Legal and Ethical Issues in Emergency Medicine

T0202241

What Do I Do Now? Emergency Medicine

SERIES EDITORS-IN-CHIEF

Catherine A. Marco, MD, FACEP
Professor, Emergency Medicine & Surgery
Wright State University Boonshoft School of Medicine
Dayton, Ohio

OTHER VOLUMES IN THE SERIES

Pediatric Medical Emergencies
Pediatric Traumatic Emergencies

FORTHCOMING VOLUMES

Critical Care Emergencies

Legal and Ethical Issues in Emergency Medicine

Edited by

Eileen F. Baker, MD, PhD, FACEP
Assistant Professor
University of Toledo College of Medicine and Life Sciences
Toledo, Ohio
Riverwood Emergency Services, Inc.
Perrysburg, Ohio

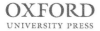

OXFORD
UNIVERSITY PRESS

OXFORD
UNIVERSITY PRESS

Oxford University Press is a department of the University of Oxford. It furthers
the University's objective of excellence in research, scholarship, and education
by publishing worldwide. Oxford is a registered trade mark of Oxford University
Press in the UK and certain other countries.

Published in the United States of America by Oxford University Press
198 Madison Avenue, New York, NY 10016, United States of America.

Library of Congress Cataloging-in-Publication Data
Names: Baker, Eileen F., editor.
Title: Legal and ethical issues in emergency medicine / edited by Eileen F. Baker.
Other titles: What do I do now?
Description: New York, NY : Oxford University Press, [2020] |
Series: What do I do now? |
Includes bibliographical references and index.
Identifiers: LCCN 2019052449 (print) | LCCN 2019052450 (ebook) |
ISBN 9780190066420 (paperback) | ISBN 9780190066444 (epub) | ISBN 9780190066451
Subjects: MESH: Emergency Medicine—legislation & jurisprudence |
Emergency Medicine—ethics | Case Reports
Classification: LCC RC86.95 (print) | LCC RC86.95 (ebook) |
NLM WB 33.1 | DDC 174.2/96025—dc23
LC record available at https://lccn.loc.gov/2019052449
LC ebook record available at https://lccn.loc.gov/2019052450

This material is not intended to be, and should not be considered, a substitute for medical or other
professional advice. Treatment for the conditions described in this material is highly dependent on
the individual circumstances. And, while this material is designed to offer accurate information with
respect to the subject matter covered and to be current as of the time it was written, research and
knowledge about medical and health issues is constantly evolving and dose schedules for medications
are being revised continually, with new side effects recognized and accounted for regularly. Readers
must therefore always check the product information and clinical procedures with the most up-to-date
published product information and data sheets provided by the manufacturers and the most recent
codes of conduct and safety regulation. The publisher and the authors make no representations or
warranties to readers, express or implied, as to the accuracy or completeness of this material. Without
limiting the foregoing, the publisher and the authors make no representations or warranties as to the
accuracy or efficacy of the drug dosages mentioned in the material. The authors and the publisher do
not accept, and expressly disclaim, any responsibility for any liability, loss, or risk that may be claimed
or incurred as a consequence of the use and/or application of any of the contents of this material.

9 8 7 6 5 4 3 2 1
Printed by Marquis, Canada

Contents

Preface

Emergency physicians encounter challenging situations on a daily basis. In fact, it is the challenging nature of this work that appeals to its practitioners. While many clinical presentations place demands on the physician's medical knowledge, often the source of greatest angst results from nonmedical conflict. Yet, physicians can feel unprepared for the social, political, legal, and ethical dilemmas they face. All practitioners learn, over time, to navigate the waters of difficult cases. This book is intended to provide additional insight into some of the toughest legal and ethical quandaries that emergency physicians encounter.

Each chapter begins with a clinical vignette, focusing on an important legal or ethical dilemma that emergency physicians face, ending with the query: "What do you do now?" What follows is a discussion of the topic at hand, presented in a manner similar to "curbsiding" a colleague with expertise in the area. The case concludes with a summary of recommendations, as well as Key Points to remember and Suggested Reading, should the reader desire supplementary information.

It is my hope that readers can add to their "bag of tricks" by gaining foresight into legal and ethical pitfalls, thereby avoiding potentially problematic situations in their clinical practice.

Contributors

Jay M. Brenner, MD
Associate Professor
Department of Emergency
  Medicine
SUNY-Upstate Medical University,
  Syracuse, NY, USA

Arthur R. Derse, MD, JD, FACEP
Center for Bioethics and Medical
  Humanities, and Department of
  Emergency Medicine
Medical College of Wisconsin
Milwaukee, WI, USA

Diane L. Gorgas, MD
Professor—Clinical, Vice Chair of
  Academic Affairs
Department of Emergency
  Medicine, Executive Director,
  Office of Global Health
The Ohio State University
  Wexner Medical Center, The
  Ohio State University College
  of Medicine
Columbus, OH, USA

**Purva Grover, MD,
MBA, FACEP**
Medical Director
Pediatric Emergency Department,
  Emergency Services
  Institute, Cleveland Clinic
Cleveland, OH, USA

**Kenneth V. Iserson, MD, MBA,
FACEP, FAAEM, FIFEM**
Professor Emeritus
Department of Emergency
  Medicine
The University of Arizona
Tucson, AZ, USA

**Chadd K. Kraus, DO, DrPH,
MPH, FACEP**
Director
Emergency Medicine Research; Core
  Faculty, Emergency Medicine
  Residency
Danville, PA, USA

Simiao Li-Sauerwine, MD, MS
Assistant Professor—Clinical,
  Assistant Residency Program
  Director
Department of Emergency
  Medicine
The Ohio State University Wexner
  Medical Center
Columbus, OH, USA

Catherine A. Marco, MD
Professor
Department of Emergency
  Medicine
Wright State University Boonshoft
  School of Medicine, Attending
  Physician, Miami Valley Hospital
Dayton, OH, USA

Shannon Markus, MD, MPH
Department of Emergency
  Medicine
Vanderbilt University Medical
  Center
Nashville, TN, USA

Jillian L. McGrath, MD
Associate Professor
Department of Emergency Medicine
The Ohio State University Wexner
  Medical Center
Columbus, OH, USA

Kelsey Nestor, MD
Department of Emergency Medicine
Vanderbilt University Medical
  Center
Nashville, TN, USA

Thomas E. Robey, MD, PhD
Assistant Clinical Professor
Elson S. Floyd School of Medicine
Washington State University,
  Providence Regional Medical
  Center
Everett, WA, USA

Lydia M. Sahlani, MD
Assistant Professor
Department of Emergency Medicine
The Ohio State University Wexner
  Medical Center
Columbus, OH, USA

Markayle R. Schears, BS
Nanjing University-Johns Hopkins
  University Graduate Program,
  UW-Madison
Bachelor of Science
Madison, WI, USA

**Raquel M. Schears, MD,
MPH, MBA**
UCF Professor
Department of Emergency
  Medicine
Osceola Regional Medical Center
Orlando, FL, USA

Ahmed Shaikh, MD
Emergency Medicine Residency
NewYork-Presbyterian
New York, NY, USA

Jeremy R. Simon, MD, PhD
Department of Emergency
  Medicine
Columbia University
New York, NY, USA

Robert C. Solomon, MD, FACEP
Medical Director
Emergency Department, Medical
  Director, Hospitalist Service,
  Ellwood City Medical Center
Ellwood City, PA, USA

Arvind Venkat, MD
Department of Emergency
   Medicine
Allegheny Health Network
Pittsburgh, PA, USA

Carmen Wolfe, MD
Department of Emergency
   Medicine
Vanderbilt University Medical
   Center
Nashville, TN, USA

Sara R. Zaidi, MD
Emergency Medicine Residency
NewYork-Presbyterian
New York, NY, USA

Alexander Zoretich, MD
Department of Emergency
   Medicine
Allegheny Health Network
Pittsburgh, PA, USA

1 "Send Me the Pictures"

Catherine A. Marco

A 38-year-old man presents to the emergency department
(ED) following a dog bite to the face. The wound extends
through the entire upper lip, cheek, and lower eyelid. You
are concerned for lacrimal duct involvement. You call the
plastic surgeon on call. He requests that you send a text
with photographs so he can determine the plan of action.
Can you text patient photographs? Is permission required?
What safeguards should be used to protect patient
confidentiality?

What do you do now?

PRIVACY AND CONFIDENTIALITY IN THE
EMERGENCY DEPARTMENT

Confidentiality is an important topic in the ED, where the environment is often loud and chaotic. The importance of confidentiality in medicine has been recognized for centuries. The Hippocratic Oath (circa 400 BC) states in part: "All that may come to my knowledge in the exercise of my profession or in daily commerce with men, which ought not to be spread abroad, I will keep secret and will never reveal." Similarly, in modern times, the American Medical Association (AMA) Principles of Ethics states, "A physician shall respect the rights of patients, colleagues, and other health professionals, and shall safeguard patient confidences and privacy within the constraints of the law."

Emergency physicians have a duty to protect patient confidentiality, within the constraints of the law. It is an ethical and legal duty and serves to maintain patient trust and protects patients' relationships, employment, and personal desire for confidentiality of medical information. However, the duty to keep records confidential is not absolute. There are specific circumstances where confidentiality should appropriately be breached, including judicial proceedings, public reporting statutes, and in cases where patients or other parties are in danger.

The ED environment poses specific questions and challenges. The environment may be loud or crowded, or present conditions where others may see or overhear personal information. Reportable diseases are often encountered. Interested parties may telephone to inquire about patients. Patients or visitors may wish to record procedures or interactions for personal records. Providers may wish to film or record interesting cases for educational purposes.

The Health Insurance Portability and Accountability Act of 1996 (HIPAA) Privacy Rule protects all "individually identifiable health information" held or transmitted by a covered entity or its business associate, in any form or media, whether electronic, paper, or oral. The Privacy Rule calls this information protected health information (PHI) (Table 1.1).

A covered entity may use and disclose PHI for its own treatment, payment, and health care operations activities. *Health care operations* include quality assessment and improvement, case management, care coordination,

TABLE 1.1 **Protected Health Information**

1. Names

2. All geographical subdivisions smaller than a state, including street address, city, county, precinct, zip code

3. All elements of dates (except year) for dates directly related to an individual, including birth date, admission date, discharge date, date of death; and all ages over 89

4. Phone numbers

5. Fax numbers

6. Electronic mail addresses

7. Social Security numbers

8. Medical record numbers

9. Health plan beneficiary numbers

10. Account numbers

11. Certificate/license numbers

12. Vehicle identifiers and serial numbers, including license plate numbers

13. Device identifiers and serial numbers

14. Web Universal Resource Locators (URLs)

15. Internet Protocol (IP) address numbers

16. Biometric identifiers, including finger- and voiceprints

17. Full-face photographic images and any comparable images

18. Any other unique identifying number, characteristic, or code

competency assurance activities, medical reviews, audits or legal services, insurance functions, business planning, development, management, and administration. Heath care operations also include "to conduct training programs in which students, trainees, or practitioners in areas of health care learn under supervision to practice or improve their skills as health care providers." Of note, the Privacy Rule includes no restrictions on the use or disclosure of de-identified health information.

ELECTRONIC MEDIA AND DISSEMINATION OF INFORMATION

Electronic communications have made dissemination of information incredibly easy and have raised important questions about the appropriate and inappropriate use of patient information. The Conversation Prism displays the vast extent and interactions of electronic media (Figure 1.1).

Electronic media may be appropriately used within medicine for communication and education. It may also be fraught with peril when communications or social media posts include PHI, derogatory comments, or inappropriate personal information.

The American College of Emergency Physicians (ACEP) has a policy "Confidentiality of Patient Information." It emphasizes that all physicians have an ethical and legal duty to guard and respect the confidential nature of the personal information conveyed during the patient-physician encounter. "Emergency physicians implicitly promise to preserve confidentiality of patient information, a promise that in turn promotes patients' autonomy and trust in their emergency physicians."

Individual assessment of clinical circumstances is encouraged in cases involving minors, drug testing, employee health, perpetrators and victims of violent crimes, medical records, the media, and communicable and sexually transmitted diseases. "In such cases not directly addressed by the law, individualized assessment and management, based on these principles of confidentiality of patient information, constitute best practice."

The American Medical Association has stated

> The internet has created the ability for medical students and physicians to communicate and share information quickly and to reach millions of people easily. Participating in social networking and other similar opportunities can support physicians' personal expression, enable individual physicians to have a professional presence online, foster collegiality and camaraderie within the profession, provide opportunities to widely disseminate public health messages and other health communication. Social networks, blogs, and other forms of communication online also create new challenges to the patient-physician relationship.

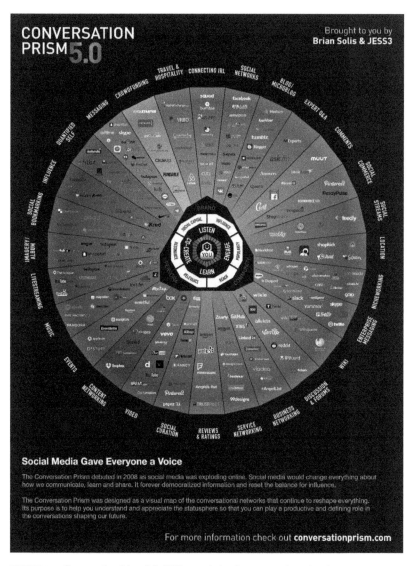

FIGURE 1.1 Conversation Prism 5.0. (With permission for conversation prism.)

In addition to legal consideration under the HIPAA Privacy Rule, safeguards should be considered when using electronic communications. PHI should not be included without express patient consent. Many institutions have secure electronic servers for transmission of confidential patient information.

FILMING OF PATIENTS AND STAFF

Filming of patients, visitors, and staff in the ED environment is a controversial topic. Most ED staff are opposed to filming of any type, and many institutions have policies prohibiting filming by patients and visitors. However, such policies are difficult to enforce, as some will record interactions surreptitiously or refuse to comply with such policies.

In their policy, "Commercial Filming of Patients in the Emergency Department," ACEP asserts that commercial filming of patients or staff may be done only if patients and staff give fully informed consent prior to filming.

> Because commercial filming cannot benefit a patient medically and may compromise both their privacy and confidentiality, filming should not commence unless and until a patient with full, unencumbered decision making capacity can explicitly consent or, if institutional policies permit surrogate consent for commercial filming, that consent is given. Patients who do consent should have the right to rescind their consent up until a reasonable time before broadcast to the public.

ACEP also calls on hospitals to develop and implement policies to regulate commercial filming that are approved by hospital governing bodies and approved by hospital ethics committees (or their representatives), "which should ideally include physicians and community members."

ETHICAL CONSIDERATIONS

Autonomy

Respect for patient autonomy refers to respect for an individual's right to make medical decisions about his or her own body. Providers should respect the right of patients to make medical decisions that reflect their own goals and values. Decisions should be based on clear and accurate information and should be free of coercion. Patient images containing PHI may only be disseminated with the patient's express permission. With patient permission, electronic communications for patient care can improve rapid access to specialty care.

Beneficence

Beneficence, the obligation to act in the best interest of patients, applies to this decision. The provider has a duty to do good, or to promote the patient's welfare. In general, decisions about the use of patient information should be made with the patient's consent.

Nonmaleficence

Nonmaleficence, the obligation to not inflict harm intentionally, has application in this case. Nonmaleficence often references the phrase *primum non nocere* ("first, do no harm"). This principle mandates that the provider should avoid any action that would intentionally harm the patient. Dissemination of identifiable patient information without consent may potentially harm the patient and may erode the patient's trust in the medical profession.

CASE RESOLUTION

Protected health information may be transmitted, over secure electronic servers, for patient care. Patient consent should be obtained, and PHI should be limited to the minimum necessary information. Some institutions use a secure, HIPAA-compliant texting system. If available, this system should be used to ensure privacy and delivery only to the designated provider. If not available at your institution, it is not recommended to send an identifiable photograph by nonsecure technology. Alternatives include a verbal description of the wound, and the surgeon should arrive in person to provide consultative services.

You explain to the plastic surgeon that you do not have a secure means of transmitting the photos from your institution, and that you do not feel comfortable sending the images. After describing the extent of the wounds, the surgeon agrees to see the patient in your ED.

KEY POINTS TO REMEMBER

- Keep PHI confidential.
- PHI may be appropriately disseminated electronically for patient care, with patient consent.
- PHI may be disclosed as required by law for reportable diseases or for judicial proceedings.
- PHI may be disclosed if a patient or third party is in danger.
- PHI may be appropriately used for educational purposes.

Suggested Reading

45 CFR 164.501. Uses and disclosures of protected health information: General rules. https://www.govregs.com/regulations/expand/title45_chapterA_part164_subpartE_section164.502. Accessed February 26, 2019.

American College of Emergency Physicians. Clinical policy: commercial filming of patients in the emergency department. Available at https://www.acep.org/patient-care/policy-statements/commercial-filming-of-patients-in-the-emergency-department/#sm.0000lu36v11cvufjysh9ltlknlyc0. Revised June 2015 with current title. Accessed February 26, 2019.

American College of Emergency Physicians. Clinical policy: confidentiality of patient information. Available at: https://www.acep.org/patient-care/policy-statements/confidentiality-of-patient-information/. Revised January 2017 with current title. Accessed April 5, 2019.

American College of Emergency Physicians. Use of social media by emergency physicians. Available at: https://www.acep.org/patient-care/policy-statements/use-of-social-media-by-emergency-physicians/#sm.0000lu36v11cvufjysh9ltlknlyc0. Approved September 2018. Accessed February 19, 2019.

American College of Emergency Physicians. Confidentiality of patient information. https://www.acep.org/patient-care/policy-statements/confidentiality-of-patient-information/#sm.0000lu36v11cvufjysh9ltlknlyc0. Revised January 2017 with current title. Accessed February 19, 2019

American Medical Association. Professionalism in the use of social media. Available at: https://www.ama-assn.org/delivering-care/ethics/professionalism-use-social-media. Accessed February 26, 2019.

Ben-Assuli O. Electronic health records, adoption, quality of care, legal and privacy issues and their implementation in emergency departments. *Health Policy*. 2015 Mar;119(3):287–297.

Carley S, Beardsell I, May N, et al. Social-media-enabled learning in emergency medicine: a case study of the growth, engagement and impact of a free open access medical education blog. *Postgrad Med J*. 2018 Feb;94(1108):92–96.

Langdorf MI, Lin M. Emergency medicine scholarship in the digital age. *West J Emerg Med*. 2016 Sep;17(5):511–512.

US Department of Health and Human Services. Summary of the HIPAA Privacy Rule. https://www.hhs.gov/hipaa/for-professionals/privacy/laws-regulations/index.html. Content last reviewed July 26, 2013. Accessed February 26, 2019.

2 Why We Care for Anyone with Anything at Anytime

Jay M. Brenner

A 7-year-old girl presents to the emergency department (ED) at Hospital A with her mother, complaining of a suspected sexual assault by the girl's father. Hospital A is the only hospital in the city with a pediatric ED and a pediatric Sexual Assault Nurse Examiner (SANE) program. The mother is pregnant with twins at 32 weeks' gestation. During triage, she begins to have contractions spaced 5 minutes apart and requests to leave with her daughter to go to Hospital B, about a mile away, to be checked for labor. There is no one available to stay with her daughter. The grandmother lives 5 hours away and is on her way. Hospital A, where you work, does not have a labor and delivery unit; however, it does have an obstetric/gynecological (OB/GYN) service. They cover for gynecological emergencies and arrange for and accept immediate transfer to another immediately adjacent Hospital C for obstetrical emergencies. The mother prefers to go to Hospital B where her OB/GYN has privileges.

What do you do now?

EMERGENCY MEDICAL TREATMENT AND ACTIVE LABOR ACT AND DEFERRED CARE

To decide what to do in this complicated situation, the emergency physician (EP) should apply the rapid decision-making model (see Figure 2.1). First, clearly the Emergency Medical Treatment and Active Labor Act (EMTALA) applies. Second, try to find an option that will buy you time to deliberate without causing excessive risk to the patient. The girl can wait to have a forensic SANE examination after having a medical screening exam (MSE) provided there are no emergency medical conditions identified; the woman, however, cannot wait to be checked for labor. Third, consider if it passes the following tests:

1. Impartiality Test: What if you were the patient(s)? The girl would not want to have a forensic SANE examination without her mother or another trusted family member present. The woman would like to be checked for active labor by an OB/GYN physician that she trusts. She would prefer to have her OB/GYN physician.

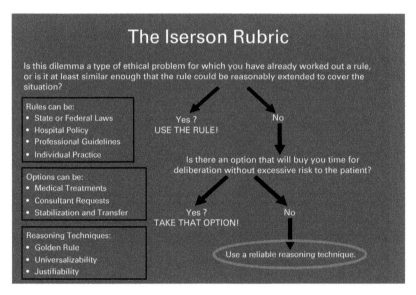

FIGURE 2.1 The Iserson Rubric

2. Universality Test: Would you approve other physicians all acting the same? Other physicians might suggest that you should attempt to persuade the woman to be checked for active labor as quickly as possible by a qualified OB/GYN provider and to keep the girl in the ED until her forensic SANE examination could be completed and her safe disposition could be ensured.

3. Interpersonal Justifiability Test: Are there good reasons to justify your course of action? Yes, the girl should not have to undergo the trauma of the forensic SANE examination without her mother or another trusted family member such as her maternal grandmother present. Also, the woman should not have to worry about her insurance covering her obstetrical triage evaluation at Hospital C immediately adjacent to Hospital A, nor should she have to worry about the quality of the care provided. If she insists on going to Hospital B for evaluation of active labor, then she should be permitted to leave, and Hospital A should make reasonable transportation accommodations in spite of concerns for untoward events such as precipitous delivery of premature infants. For this very reason though, the EP should make every effort to convince the woman to stay short of coercion.

EMTALA

Fortunately, the case presented above has a well-demarcated law that applies to the given situation, and this law has spawned multiple policies in hospitals in order to comply with the law. EMTALA became law in the United States in 1986 to address a problem of patient dumping: private hospitals were turning away patients who were uninsured or underinsured. EMTALA requires the following:

1. Any individual who comes and requests emergency care based on the prudent layperson standard must receive a MSE from a qualified medical personnel (QMP) to determine whether an emergency medical condition exists. Examination and treatment cannot be delayed to inquire about methods of payment or insurance coverage. EDs also must post signs that notify patients and visitors of their rights to a MSE and treatment.

2. If an emergency medical condition exists, treatment must be provided until the emergency medical condition is resolved or stabilized. If the hospital does not have the capability to treat the emergency medical condition, an "appropriate" transfer of the patient to another hospital must be done in accordance with the EMTALA provisions.

3. Hospitals with specialized capabilities are obligated to accept transfers from hospitals that lack the capability to treat unstable emergency medical conditions.

A QMP is a provider who has the ability to perform a MSE, including a physician, physician assistant, nurse practitioner, or midwife. The Center for Medicare and Medicaid Services (CMS) requires hospitals to report violations of any components of EMTALA to CMS. The Health and Human Services Office of the Inspector General (OIG) investigates these complaints and holds hospitals and physicians accountable to a $50,000 fine if they are found to be in violation. This is in spite of the mandate being unfunded, or at least vastly underfunded.

Examples of Violations

It may help the reader to consider examples of EMTALA violations to help understand when EMTALA does and does not apply. The OIG fined hospitals as opposed to physicians in 96% of the 196 violations from 2002 to 2015 that were imposed. The OIG fined individual physicians in only 4% of the cases. The only EP to receive a fine refused to perform a MSE on an adolescent girl who was pregnant because the EP erroneously thought that the 17-year-old girl was unable to consent to treatment for a reproductive health complaint of abdominal pain, vaginal bleeding, and perirectal numbness in Louisiana. The other fined physicians included two obstetricians, two surgeons, an orthopedic surgeon, a neurosurgeon, and an ophthalmologist, who all either refused to evaluate and treat an ED patient where they were on call or refused a transfer.

While violations against individual physicians are rare, EPs should still concern themselves with violations against hospitals where they work. From 2002 to2013, 88.5% of 166 violations were for failure to provide an appropriate MSE or stabilizing treatment. Twelve percent were for refusal to

TABLE 2.1 **Sample EMTALA Violations Secondary to Delay to be Seen**

Chief Complaint	Time to Be Seen	Outcome
Abnormal hemoglobin	7 hours	Died in ED
Chest pain	3 hours	Died outside of ED
Shortness of breath	40 minutes	Left against medical advice (AMA)
Acute appendicitis	1.5 hours	Surgery at another hospital

accept an appropriate transfer; 5% were for on-call physicians failing to respond to a request to evaluate and treat an ED patient. The first category includes patients who experienced exceptionally long delays (see Table 2.1) and insufficient stabilization prior to discharge (see Table 2.2).

CASE RESOLUTION

Ultimately, the woman agreed to be transferred to Hospital C immediately adjacent to Hospital A by wheelchair through a sky tunnel. She left her daughter in the care of the pediatric ED staff, and a child life specialist accompanied the girl until her maternal grandmother arrived from out of state to chaperone the forensic SANE exam. The woman, pregnant with twins, was found to be in false labor at Hospital C and was discharged in time to take her daughter home from Hospital A, separately from the father accused of molestation.

TABLE 2.2 **Sample EMTALA Violations Secondary to Lack of Stabilization**

Discharge Diagnosis	Ultimate Diagnosis	Outcome
Hunger pains	Gastric hemorrhage	Death
Inability to walk	Acetabular fracture	Surgery
Heroin overdose	Heroin overdose	Death
Knee pain	Respiratory failure	Death
Scapula fracture	Rib and back fractures	Surgery

- EMTALA requires EPs to perform an MSE on all patients seeking emergency care and to stabilize any emergency medical conditions identified.
- EPs must arrange for appropriate transfer when they do not have access to the necessary specialist.
- EPs must accept appropriate transfers when they and their hospital have the capability and capacity to accommodate the request being made.
- Violations of EMTALA may result in a fine to the hospital or the individual physician.

Suggested Reading

American College of Emergency Physicians. EMTALA fact sheet. https://www.acep.org/life-as-a-physician/ethics--legal/emtala/emtala-fact-sheet/. Accessed March 3, 2019.

Bitterman, RA. EMTALA and the ethical delivery of hospital emergency services. *Emerg Med Clin N Am.* 2006;*24*(3):557–577.

Brenner, JM. Do prosecuted EMTALA cases actually reflect our duty to care? *Empire State Epic.* 2014:11–13.

Iserson, KV. Ethical principles—emergency medicine. *Emerg Med Clin N Am.* 2006;*24*(3):515–545.

Terp, S, Wang, B, Raffetto, B, et al. Individual physician penalties resulting from violation of Emergency Medical Treatment and Labor Act: a review of Office of the Inspector General Patient Dumping Settlements, 2002–2015. *Acad Emerg Med.* April 2017;*4*(24):422–446.

3 No and Yes

Kenneth V. Iserson

A 50-year-old woman comes into the emergency department (ED) with sudden, severe, dull/aching pain in her right shoulder for 1 hour. She denies prior pain, injury, arthritis, or neck pain. Further history and review of systems are unremarkable. She smokes. She appears to have moderate pain but an unremarkable physical examination. Her electrocardiogram (ECG) demonstrates an acute anterolateral myocardial infarction (MI). She has a normal chest X-ray and elevated troponin.

You explain that she needs an immediate cardiac catheterization. You hand her the consent form and offer to answer questions. She says, "No, I just want to leave." You ask, "Do you understand how serious a heart attack is?" and leave, frustrated. Her nurse enters and talks with her, before summoning you into the room. "Ask her to sign the consent again." The patient signs it. "What did you say to her?" you ask. "That she would die without the cath," she says.

You now have a refusal followed by a possibly coerced consent. You question if the patient has the capacity to refuse or agree.

What do you do now?

ASSESSMENT OF DECISION-MAKING CAPACITY

Physicians must assess patients' decision-making capacity to know whether to follow their directions about their medical care or to implement an advance directive or employ surrogate decision-makers. In doing this, emergency physicians (EPs) try to balance their respect for the patient's self-determination with their concern for his or her well-being. Respect for patient self-determination is the basis of the moral and legal right to refuse or accept treatment, even life-saving treatment. Patient autonomy, as described by Justice Benjamin Cardozo, means "Every human being of adult years and sound mind has a right to determine what shall be done with his own body" [Schoendorff v. Society of New York Hosp., 105 N.E. 92, 93 (N.Y. 1914)]. However, only those with decisional capacity have this right. The right is further limited by the need to protect others from harm, such as not allowing patients with highly communicable diseases to refuse isolation or treatment.

The presumption for most adult patients is that they have decision-making capacity unless they are severely cognitively disabled, comatose, or have significantly altered mental status. Clinicians generally only question patients' decision-making capacity when they refuse recommended medical interventions or otherwise make what is considered an abnormal decision. However, disagreeing with a clinician's recommended healthcare interventions does not mean the patient lacks decision-making capacity, but may only signal a difference between the goals and values of the provider and those of the patient. It's unclear how often clinicians proceed with intervention in patients that do not oppose them but lack decision-making capacity.

Decision-making capacity differs from competence, which is a legal term and generally determined by a court. If a court has deemed a person incompetent, they will appoint a guardian to make some or all the person's decisions.

For their patients, EPs must quickly make the determination of decision-making capacity. Unless it is the institution's policy, psychiatrists or other specialist generally do not accept this task. While a lack of capacity is obvious in the unconscious or delirious patient, it often is less apparent when the patient remains verbal and at least somewhat coherent. Due to the time-sensitive nature of many emergency medicine (EM) interventions, consultation, such as from the institutional bioethics committee, may be unavailable.

When doing these evaluations, EPs must recognize conditions that do not automatically preclude decision-making capacity. These include advanced age; intoxication from medications, drugs, or alcohol; neurological deficits; diminished cognitive capabilities; and communication problems (language or speech). Decision-making capacity can wax and wane, depending on the patient's condition. Sometimes, medical interventions, such as administering antidotes, providing oxygen, or relieving acute pain can improve the patient's decision-making capacity. Many clinicians mistakenly equate a mental status exam (orientation, memory, attention, and reasoning ability) with decisional capacity; that is not accurate. Those with a normal mental status exam do not necessarily have decisional capacity for the healthcare decision in question. Likewise, patients with an abnormal mental status may, on occasion, be found decisional, depending on assessing the elements that follow.

To assess patients' decision-making capacity, the EP must discover whether they (1) understand the healthcare options as presented to them, (2) understand the risks and benefits of each of those options, and (3) choose an option consistent with their stable value system. Asking patients why they selected an option can elicit information about their choice's relation to their value system. While this process may slightly extend the consent process, it is valuable for the patient to be able to clarify available choices and for clinicians to gain patient trust and provide true informed consent.

Decision-making capacity is decision relative. Decisional capacity relates to both the complexity of the decision and the probability of harm to the patient. A patient may have the capacity to make some decisions that are relatively simple, and the risks are minimal. The same patient may lack the capacity to make other decisions that require processing complex information and where a bad decision carries great risk. We recognize that easily when dealing with children. For example, while a 5-year-old may have the capacity to choose food options from a menu, it's doubtful that she has the capacity to drive a car. Higher standards are employed for decisions with greater complexity (e.g., decision about how to proceed with diagnosing a possible pulmonary embolus) and more serious/irreversible outcomes (e.g., whether to have a cardiac catheterization for an acute myocardial infarction [AMI]).

Having the capacity to make a specific decision involves more than simply stating a preference for or against a treatment option. Rather, capacity means that the patient must articulate a knowledge of the options available (as described by the clinician), an awareness of the risks and benefits (as they see them) of the options, and how their value system led them to make the choice they made. The first two of these are a standard part of the informed consent process, asking the patient to explain what they were told. Without this knowledge, there is no informed consent. The last element, why they made the decision they did, is the crux of the process. It provides insight into the patient's thought process and may indicate a need for further clarification or that the decision is outside his or her normal value system. Note that some religious objections to standard treatment (not accepting blood products, e.g.) may reasonably fall within a person's normal value system. However, using this process allows the clinician an opportunity to clarify possible adverse outcomes for the patient.

It's now obvious that determining decision-making capacity in a situation that poses significant risk to the patient may be difficult. As Buchanan (1995, p. 63) wrote,

> How high we set the threshold of competence here . . . depends upon how we balance competing considerations. How willing are we to allow some individuals to suffer avoidable harm in an attempt to respect their rights of self-determination? How willing are we to allow some individuals to suffer avoidable harm to prevent others from having defective choices made for them? Although there is no magic formula for setting the threshold of competence for a particular type of decision, it is possible to identify the most important factors that should be taken into account for such a determination. Perhaps the most important of these are the probability and the magnitude of harm occurring as a result of respecting the patient's choice.

CASE RESOLUTION

In this patient's case, we start over by asking the patient about what options for treatment she has. If she doesn't know them, explain them (again). Describe the risks and benefits, although it's best not to use the "you're going to die" card unless it is certain. Ask her to describe them back in her own words. Then ask if she wants to proceed with the catheterization, as she previously suggested. If so, ask why. You may also want to ask why she initially refused. That may raise other concerns that can be addressed.

KEY POINTS TO REMEMBER

- Decision-making capacity (rather than "competence," a legal term) is the ability to make decisions about one's own medical care.
- Having decision-making capacity rests on the patients understanding of their healthcare options and choosing an option consistent with their stable value system.
- Capacity is decision relative, meaning that the criteria to have decisional capacity depend on the complexity of the decision and the seriousness of possible outcomes.
- Individuals can have fluctuating decision-making capacity.

Suggested Reading

Buchanan AE. The question of competence. In: Iserson KV, Sanders AB, Mathieu DR (eds.), *Ethics in Emergency Medicine*, 2nd edition. Tucson, AZ: Galen Press; 1995:63–67.

Iserson KV. Principles of medical ethics. In: Marco C, Schears R (eds.), *Ethical Dilemmas in Emergency Medicine*. New York: Cambridge University Press; 2015:1–17.

Iserson KV, Heine C. Bioethics. In: Walls RM, Hockberger RS, Gausche-Hill M, et al. (eds.), *Rosen's Emergency Medicine: Concepts and Clinical Practice*, 9th edition. Philadelphia: Mosby; 2017: Chapter 10e.

4 "Thanks, But No Thanks!"

Arthur R. Derse

A 45-year-old male comes to the emergency department (ED) with severe chest pain and smelling of alcohol, though lacking obvious signs of intoxication. No one accompanies him. Vital signs are normal, except for a pulse of 120. Initial electrocardiogram (ECG shows 1-mm ST depressions in II, III, and aVF. He is given oxygen and nitroglycerin, which relieves his pain. A second ECG and his vital signs all are normal. A chest x-ray is normal. When the patient is asked about drug use, he doesn't answer. He asks if his blood has been tested for drugs. The ED physician explains, "Yes, that's routine for severe chest pain." The patient says he no longer has chest pain and refuses further treatment, saying he does not want any tests done and asks to be discharged. He appears to have decision-making capacity. His laboratory tests are being run, but have not yet been reported, and the ED physician is uncertain if an order to cancel the alcohol level and drug screens were to be made, it would be in time to stop the processes.

What do you do now?

REFUSAL OF DIAGNOSIS AND TREATMENT

The problem of patients who refuse diagnostic workup or medical treatment for serious symptoms or signs can be a potentially high-stakes problem for the ED physician, as a patient who refuses diagnosis or treatment may encounter subsequent morbidity and mortality. As well, physicians generally have a duty to provide the standard of care for diagnosis and treatment of the patient's complaints. Falling below the standard of care may result in liability for damages. This duty correlates with the bioethical principles of beneficence (the duty to act to benefit the patient) and nonmaleficence (the duty not to harm patients).

Patients may refuse diagnostic measures and medical treatment for many reasons. Some of these may be well-considered decisions that are aligned with the patient's values. However, patients also may be affected by factors or concerns that may be seemingly of less importance than the health care concerns that brought the patient to the ED (either by their own will or by others) in the first place. Even more perplexing, patients may not disclose the reasons that they now are refusing diagnosis or treatment. Nothing can be more frustrating to the busy emergency physician than this sudden derangement of what is usually an alignment of physician and patient goals, namely, to accurately diagnose and effectively treat the patient's symptoms or medical problems.

Adding to the complexity of this problem is that, in the United States, patients have the legal right to refuse treatment, including life-sustaining medical treatment with some exceptions (e.g., loss of decision-making capacity due to suicidal ideation or in the case of an emergency when the patient lacks decision-making capacity and no one is legally authorized to speak for the patient). This right to refuse treatment is one that is grounded in law first established over a century ago with *Schloendorff v. Society of New York Hospital*: the principle that decisions to undergo medical treatment shall be made by the adult of sound mind—and not merely because a physician's professional judgment indicated that an intervention was required. The subsequent landmark case of *Salgo v. Leland Stanford Jr. Board of Trustees* established that not only did the physician need the consent of the patient but also the consent needed to be an informed one. This information should include the nature of the procedure, the risks and side effects, and the alternatives, including what would happen if there were no treatment. In some states, the standard of the information to be disclosed is that which the average prudent practitioner would disclose, while in others, the standard is that information that a reasonable (objective) patient would want to know. This doctrine was further expanded in another landmark case, *Truman v. Thomas,* that required that a patient's refusal needed to be accompanied by an offer to explain the consequences of that refusal. If the patient refused but was not informed of the potential consequences of the refusal, the physician may be liable for the consequences.

The patient's right to refuse treatment, including life-sustaining medical treatment, has been established over the past half century. Years ago, a patient who might refuse a life-sustaining transfusion (e.g., on religious grounds) might be seen as suicidal, and therefore the patient's decision could be overridden with a forced transfusion. In more recent years, patients have won the right to refuse not only blood transfusions but also life-sustaining medical treatment in the form of ventilators, feeding tubes, resuscitation, and dialysis. Patients now have a very strong legal ground for refusal, a liberty interest, grounded in the Fourteenth Amendment due process clause of the US Constitution. This right is not unlimited. For instance, patients may not have the right to refuse detainment and treatment if they are a danger to themselves or others, but they may be able to refuse psychotropic medications being forced on them.

Since patients who refuse life-sustaining medical treatment—or the diagnosis and workup of symptoms and signs that may result in grave circumstances—the decision to refuse recommended medical diagnosis and treatment should be a carefully considered one. Essential to these types of refusals is the principle that the patient who refuses must have the decisional capability to do so. Patients who lack decision-making capacity are unable to evaluate the consequences of their refusal and thus cannot make an informed refusal.

Decision-making capacity determination should be a skill possessed by all emergency practitioners. In some cases, psychiatric or neuropsychological consultation maybe required, but in most cases the examination to determine decision-making capacity is able to be performed without mental health specialty expertise. The standard for decision-making capacity is that the patient is able to understand the information, to weigh the information

against the patient's set of values, to come to a decision, and to communicate that decision to the emergency practitioner. The decision should also
(eventually) be consistent over time.

Physicians have been criticized for being concerned about a patient's
capacity to make a decision only when the patient refuses, that is, not
having similar concerns about capacity when the patient agrees to the
recommended diagnosis and treatment. This may seem inconsistent.
However, since physicians recommend diagnostic measures and treatments
in the patient's best interest, when the patient refuses there is a mismatch
between the physician's understanding of the patient's interests and the
patient's differing evaluation. This difference is one that *should* engender
a conversation. The law of informed refusal requires that when the patient
refuses recommend treatment, further conversation to include an explana-
tion of consequences be offered to the patient.

If a patient refuses diagnosis and treatment of potentially serious
conditions and is unwilling to allow a determination of decision-making
capacity, the emergency practitioner has a challenging dilemma: (1) either
accept the patient's refusal and run the risk of the patient having an adverse
outcome that in retrospect was not understood as a risk and would not have
been accepted in an informed refusal or (2) persuade, cajole, or restrain the
patient involuntarily so that a determination of decision-making capacity
may be done, with a potential complaint of coercion or false imprisonment.
This dilemma is a difficult one. However, lawsuits brought by relatives and
friends of patients who died after refusal of diagnosis and treatment are
more common than suits by patients who were detained until the physician
could ensure capacity to refuse, provided this detention was made in the
least intrusive manner, and the determination was done as expeditiously as
possible. It may be easier to explain to a jury in a potential lawsuit for involuntary detention that what was done was to ensure that the patient had
the capacity to refuse, than it would be to explain to a jury why the patient's
death or severe disability was not prevented when the practitioner failed to
ensure that the patient had the basic capacity to make that decision.

The right to refuse medical treatment engenders in the emergency physician the responsibility to provide the refusing patient with the potential
consequences of the refusal, including the consequences from lack of diagnosis or treatment. This information should be provided in clear language

understandable by the patient. If the patient is willing to be informed about consequences of the refusal, the patient should express an understanding and acceptance of the consequences. In those cases where the patient has decision-making capacity and understands and waives the patient's right to be informed of the consequences of the refusal, the information should not be forced on the patient. The waiver by the decisional patient of the right to be informed of the consequences should be documented. If the patient with capacity appears to be making an informed decision to refuse, the emergency physician may consider making an attempt to enlist friends or family members who may be present with the patient (or who may be contacted with the patient's permission) to help persuade the patient to make a better decision. Emergency physicians should avoid claims that insurance will not pay for visits in which patients refuse recommended treatment since this may not be helpful and often is not accurate.

It is especially helpful to have another health care provider or other personnel available to witness the conversation that ensues from an initial refusal. Severe and common consequences of the refusal should be documented in the record and, if possible, on forms for documentation of refusal, where there is often a place for the patient's signature as a sign of understanding and acceptance (so-called against medical advice [AMA] forms). These forms may be useful but mostly serve as a signifier that the discussion has occurred. The form may not be legally protective if the refusal was not, in fact, an informed one made by a patient with the capacity to do so. The legal effect of AMA forms depends state law. The Emergency Medical Treatment and Active Labor Act (EMTALA) adds another factor. Documentation of the offer to screen for an emergent condition may be helpful should questions arise.

The standard for refusal of treatment by parents for a minor child is a very different one. Parents or guardians are to act in the best interest of their children and are generally unable to refuse life-saving treatments or necessary diagnostic procedures for serious conditions. For instance, a life-saving transfusion necessary for treatment of a child, with clear beneficial effect, is routinely supported by courts. The US Supreme Court has stated that parents are free to make martyrs of themselves but not their children. Practitioners also have duties to report suspicions of child abuse or endangerment in all jurisdictions of the United States. Parents may have more discretion for refusal when the likelihood of the benefit of diagnosis or treatment is low.

For adolescents, generally parents must give their consent for treatment, with some exceptions dictated by state statutes (e.g., sexually transmitted infection [STI] diagnosis and treatment). Adolescents who are emancipated by statute (e.g., married, living on one's own, or enlisted in the military) may make their own decisions, including refusal of life-sustaining medical treatment. In individual cases, a court may determine that the adolescent may be able to refuse life-sustaining medical treatment, and these patients may be treated similarly to adults.

CASE RESOLUTION

In this case, if the patient is willing to undergo a brief examination for decision-making capacity and the ED physician determines that the patient has capacity, does not show signs of intoxication, and is not a danger to others, then the patient may refuse continued treatment. If the laboratory tests that have already been run would be helpful to the ED physician's determination, they should be reviewed. Otherwise, the blood alcohol and drug screens should be canceled, if possible, though the physician should advocate for completing the cardiac enzymes. If, after best efforts at persuasion, the patient is still unwilling to stay and the patient understands the risks and is willing to accept them, the patient should be allowed to refuse treatment and leave, with the invitation to return when willing. This should be documented, preferably with a witness. In this case, the patient's autonomous refusal takes precedence, even if, in the emergency physician's judgment, it may result in an adverse outcome for the patient.

KEY POINTS TO REMEMBER

- Patients with decision-making capacity may accept or refuse medical treatment, including emergency medical treatment.
- Patient refusal of indicated emergency medical diagnosis and treatment that may result in significant harm to the patient should entail further discussion to determine the patient's

understanding of the reasons for the emergency physician's recommendation and the patient's understanding and acceptance of the risks of potential consequences of the refusal.

· When a patient refuses indicated emergency medical diagnosis and treatment, the emergency physician should document (1) the evaluation of the patient's capacity to make medical decisions, (2) the patient's refusal of the indicated diagnosis and treatment, (3) the offer of information about the consequences of refusal; if the patient chooses to be given that information, the emergency physician should document the understanding by the patient of the consequences of refusal.

· The patient with decision-making capacity who refuses indicated emergency medical diagnosis and treatment should be offered the opportunity to return should the patient later decide to accept diagnosis and treatment.

Suggested Reading

Alfandre D, Schumann J. What is wrong with discharges against medical advice (and how to fix them). *JAMA*. 2013;*310*(22):2393–2394.

Appelbaum PS. Assessment of patient's competence to consent to treatment. *N Engl J Med*. 2007;*357*:1834–1840.

Centers for Medicare and Medicaid Services. Emergency Medical Treatment & Labor Act (EMTALA). State operations manual appendix V—interpretive guidelines— responsibilities of Medicare participating hospitals in emergency cases. January 29, 2020, https://www.cms.gov/Regulations-and-Guidance/Legislation/EMTALA

Derse AR. What part of "no" don't you understand? Patient refusal of recommended treatment in the emergency department. *Mt Sinai J Med*. 2005;*72*(4):221–227.

Marco CM, Brenner JM, Kraus C, McGrath N, Derse AR. Refusal of emergency medical treatment: case studies and ethical foundations. *Ann Emerg Med*. 2017;*70*:696–703.

Meisel A. Legal myths about terminating life support. *Arch Intern Med*. 1991;*151*:1497–1502.

5 On the Edge of Death

Alexander Zoretich and Arvind Venkat

An elderly female rolls into the emergency department (ED) struggling to breathe, emaciated, and lethargic. She has a history of dementia and many chronic medical problems. Her respiratory status significantly declined today. A pink Physician Orders for Life-Sustaining Treatment (POLST) form stands out in color and importance among her papers. It reveals a checked box beside "CPR/Resuscitate" and "Full Treatment Measures." It was signed by the patient and doctor 3 years prior. Given this, resuscitation efforts are initiated. Despite interventions, the patient's respiratory status worsens. The patient's son arrives and states he is her next of kin and health care proxy. Despite being shown the POLST form, he states the he wants comfort measures initiated based on the patient's recent decline. He was unaware of this form and does not believe it is still valid. He says that his mother would not have wanted aggressive measures based on her living will, but he has neither this nor the health care power-of-attorney document with him.

What do you do now?

ADVANCE DIRECTIVES AND ACTIONABLE MEDICAL ORDERS

In this case, an elderly female patient with dementia presents with evidence of sepsis requiring aggressive emergency medical treatment, including intubation, central venous access, and aggressive, early antibiotic, fluid, and vasopressor treatment to have hope for survival. Accompanying her records from the nursing home where she resides is a POLST document (Figure 5.1) signed by her prior to the worsening of her cognitive state 3 years prior that indicates she wants cardiopulmonary resuscitation (CPR) should she arrest and aggressive treatment, including all of those listed, to treat an acute condition like sepsis. Her son states that the POLST form has not been updated based on her recent decline and that as her next of kin and health care power-of-attorney holder, he believes she no longer would want aggressive treatment. The emergency physician faces the dilemma of initiating either resuscitative or palliative measures in a time-constrained environment.

It is common in the ED for emergency physicians to encounter patients with end-stage or degenerative conditions where the likelihood of treatment success is poor. While there is a general default presumption to provide acute treatment given the time constraints under which emergency physicians provide care, advance directives and actionable medical orders can provide more explicit guidance as to what are the wishes of the patient in these critical circumstances. However, there is the danger that misinterpretation or misapplication can result in either undesired treatments or withholding of the same, with adverse outcomes for the patient. It therefore is important for emergency physicians to understand exactly what advance directives or actionable medical orders are and their application in the ED.

Advance directives are written documents that indicate a patient's wishes in health care, generally when facing an end-stage or degenerative condition or permanent vegetative state. These most commonly are in the form of a living will, a legal document that conforms to state-specific legislation and outlines the patient's wishes should they have an end-stage medical condition or are permanently unconscious. Often accompanying a living will is a durable health care power of attorney, another legal document with state-specific parameters that indicates whom a patient would want to make

pennsylvania DEPARTMENT OF HEALTH	Pennsylvania Orders for Life-Sustaining Treatment (POLST)	Last Name
		First/Middle Initial
		Date of Birth

FIRST follow these orders, THEN contact physician, certified registered nurse practitioner or physician assistant. This is an Order Sheet based on the person's medical condition and wishes at the time the orders were issued. Everyone shall be treated with dignity and respect.

A
Check One

CARDIOPULMONARY RESUSCITATION (CPR): Person has no pulse and is not breathing.

☐ CPR/Attempt Resuscitation ☐ DNR/Do Not Attempt Resuscitation (Allow Natural Death)

When not in cardiopulmonary arrest, follow orders in B, C and D.

B
Check One

MEDICAL INTERVENTIONS: Person has pulse and/or is breathing.

☐ **COMFORT MEASURES ONLY** Use medication by any route, positioning, wound care and other measures to relieve pain and suffering. Use oxygen, oral suction and manual treatment of airway obstruction as needed for comfort. *Do not transfer to hospital for life-sustaining treatment. Transfer if comfort needs cannot be met in current location.*

☐ **LIMITED ADDITIONAL INTERVENTIONS** Includes care described above. Use medical treatment, IV fluids and cardiac monitor as indicated. Do not use intubation, advanced airway interventions, or mechanical ventilation.

Transfer to hospital if indicated. Avoid intensive care if possible.

☐ **FULL TREATMENT** Includes care described above. Use intubation, advanced airway interventions, mechanical ventilation, and cardioversion as indicated.

Transfer to hospital if indicated. Includes intensive care.

Additional Orders _____

C
Check One

ANTIBIOTICS:

☐ No antibiotics. Use other measures to relieve symptoms.

☐ Determine use or limitation of antibiotics when infection occurs, with comfort as goal

☐ Use antibiotics if life can be prolonged

Additional Orders

D
Check One

ARTIFICIALLY ADMINISTERED HYDRATION / NUTRITION:
Always offer food and liquids by mouth if feasible

☐ No hydration and artificial nutrition by tube.

☐ Trial period of artificial hydration and nutrition by tube.

☐ Long-term artificial hydration and nutrition by tube.

Additional Orders

E
Check One

SUMMARY OF GOALS, MEDICAL CONDITION AND SIGNATURES:

Discussed with
☐ Patient
☐ Parent of Minor
☐ Health Care Agent
☐ Health Care Representative
☐ Court-Appointed Guardian
☐ Other:

Patient Goals/Medical Condition:

By signing this form, I acknowledge that this request regarding resuscitative measures is consistent with the known desires of, and in the best interest of, the individual who is the subject of the form.

Physician /PA/CRNP Printed Name:	Physician /PA/CRNP Phone Number
Physician/PA/CRNP Signature (Required):	DATE

Signature of Patient or Surrogate

Signature (required)	Name (print)	Relationship (write "self" if patient)

PADOH version 04-30-18   1 of 2

FIGURE 5.1 Physician Orders for Life-Sustaining Treatment form.

medical decisions on his or her behalf, often extending to decisions about consenting to, withholding, or withdrawing medical treatments.

For emergency physicians, there are a number of limitations and pitfalls to applying advance directives in the ED. First, patients and family members may state that they have the patient's living will or have the health care power of attorney, respectively. However, without reviewing the document itself, emergency physicians cannot assume that is the case or that what is being conveyed by a purported health care power of attorney is in alignment with the patient's wishes. Second, the assessment of whether a patient is end stage or permanently unconscious can be challenging in the short time period a patient is under the care of an emergency physician. Without such clarity, determining whether any desired limitations on medical treatment from the living will may be applicable is very challenging. Finally, state laws can place a number of limitations on the authority of health care powers of attorney to withhold or withdraw life-sustaining treatment. Emergency physicians may face medical-legal risks without consultation with legal counsel on what health care powers of attorney or next of kin can agree to on behalf of a patient in a life-and-death situation. Overall, these factors greatly limit the application of advance directives in the ED without clear evidence of a qualifying end-stage medical condition or permanent unconsciousness and careful review of the advance directive documentation, which is rarely available in this setting.

In contrast, actionable medical orders, signed by both a health care provider (physician, advance practice provider, or nurse practitioner) and a patient or surrogate decision maker, have immediate effect on execution and are meant to be portable to all health care settings. The two most common actionable medical orders encountered by emergency physicians are do not resuscitate (DNR) and POLST. The latter has become more common with the recognition that actionable medical orders should extend beyond decisions in the event of a cardiopulmonary arrest to those regarding other acute medical treatments needed to fulfill the patient's goals of care. Actionable medical orders are executed for patients in whom it would not be surprising that they might die or have severe incapacity within a 6- to 12-month period of time. Unlike previous attempts to list specific treatments, POLST documents provide orders based on goals of care: full treatment, limited treatments short of those used in intensive care, and comfort measures. The advantage of POLST documents in the ED is that their immediate application and explicit statements on what interventions are desired allows emergency physicians to readily develop treatment plans to conform to patient wishes.

However, like advance directives, actionable medical orders can lead to challenging ethical issues in the ED. While a patient with decision-making capacity always can revoke or revise their actionable medical order, the circumstances under which a surrogate decision maker can is not clear. In general, if there has been a material change in the condition of the patient, usually a further decline, it is accepted that a surrogate decision maker can override a patient-signed POLST document that indicated a desire for full treatment. It becomes more challenging when a patient with a DNR or POLST order indicating limited treatment or comfort measures may need an invasive procedure where temporary suspension of such orders would be the norm (e.g., surgery to repair a hip fracture) or when next of kin allege that such limitations no longer are congruent with the patient's wishes. In these cases, emergency physicians must assess carefully the particular clinical circumstances leading to this contradiction with the actionable medical order documentation. It is very helpful to consult with the health care provider who initiated the actionable medical order to provide context as to the goals of the patient, but this is not always possible. Those states that have regulatory or statutory recognition of POLST generally provide medical-legal protection to physicians who follow these orders in good faith.

CASE RESOLUTION

In this case, the POLST document signed by the patient indicates a desire for full treatment. However, in the 3 years since the document was signed, the patient's condition has declined to a significant degree. The patient's loving son, an involved surrogate decision maker and possibly health care power of attorney, states that the document no longer reflects the patient's condition or wishes. It therefore may be reasonable for the emergency physician to elect to initiate comfort measures in the context of a terminal event. Similarly, a default to initiating resuscitative measures to conform to the patient-signed POLST document and allow more time to explore the patient's wishes and family relationships may be reasonable as well. What are key for resolving this case are careful consideration of the patient's medical condition, review of the documentation of the patient's goals in the context of her disease, discussion with the family and ideally the outpatient provider who signed the actionable medical order, and, ultimately, synthesis of this information in a good-faith manner to uphold the values and wishes of the patient.

KEY POINTS TO REMEMBER

- Advance directives are legal documents that allow patients to outline their wishes should they be diagnosed with an end-state medical condition or permanent unconsciousness and designate a health care power of attorney empowered to make decisions on their behalf.
- Advance directives have limited application in the ED due to the time-constrained nature of patient care in this setting and the inability in that time to determine if the conditions for these documents' application are met.
- Actionable medical orders such as POLSTs are meant to be portable and have immediate application on execution.
- Actionable medical orders should be followed in good faith by emergency physicians in most circumstances, but there are times when careful review and discussion with surrogate decision makers may lead to their revision in the acute care setting.

Suggested Reading

American College of Emergency Physicians. Guidelines for emergency physicians on the interpretation of Physician Orders for Life-Sustaining Treatment (POLST). Policy statement. April 2017. https://www.acep.org/globalassets/new-pdfs/policy-statements/guidelines.emergency.physicians.on.interpretation.physician.orders.for.life-sustaining.treatment.pdf. Accessed March 23, 2019.

Jesus, JE, Geiderman, JM, Venkat, A, et al., on behalf of the American College of Emergency Physicians Ethics Committee. Physician Orders for Life-Sustaining Treatment (POLST): ethical considerations, legal issues, and emerging trends. *Ann Emerg Med.* 2014;*64*(2):140–144.

Venkat, A, Becker, J. The effect of statutory limitations on the authority of substitute decision makers on the care of patients in the intensive care unit: case examples and review of state laws affecting withdrawing or withholding life-sustaining treatment. *J Intensive Care Med.* 2014 March-April;*29*(2):71–80.

6 Who Decides?

Kenneth V. Iserson

Accompanied by her family, a 64-year-old woman presents to the emergency department (ED) with a cough and progressive weakness for 2 months, weight loss, and increasing pleuritic chest pain. Today she suddenly had hemoptysis. Her vital signs on arrival were blood pressure of 130/80 mm Hg, pulse 110, respiratory rate 22 breaths per minute, and pulse oxygen of 92% on room air. Physical examination showed a very thin woman with rales and basilar dullness bilaterally, pale mucosa, and nail clubbing. Although born abroad, she conversed easily in English and had decision-making capacity. Bedside ultrasound showed bilateral pleural effusions, and a chest x-ray confirmed large bilateral pleural effusions and a large perihilar mass. Laboratory tests showed anemia but were otherwise normal. Chest computed tomography (CT) was consistent with metastatic lung cancer. You enter her room to tell her about the diagnosis and ask about her wishes for additional interventions. She stops you and says, "Don't tell me anything. Tell my eldest son; he will make all the decisions."

What do you do now?

SURROGATE DECISION-MAKING

Patient With Decision-Making Capacity

If patients have decision-making capacity (as in this case), they can make whatever health care decisions for themselves they deem appropriate and that are within the scope of a patient's decision-making prerogatives. These health care decisions may contradict anything that is in their advance directive, including changing the person who can make their health care decisions (surrogate). They can also name adult surrogates from groups not included in the hospital policy or state statutory surrogate list. These surrogates make health care decisions for the person if they become incapacitated. As an element of patient autonomy (respect for persons), they may also, as this woman did, delegate decision-making to another adult or adults. While Western culture generally values patient autonomy and individual decision-making, much of the world and many other cultures commonly delegate their decision-making to their community, family or specific family members, or tribal or family leaders. That is what this woman did, and it should be respected.

Surrogate Decision Makers' Role

Physicians must understand surrogate decision makers' roles. In this case, it was to hear the information about his mother's case and make decisions about further treatment and diagnosis.

Information that you should supply to a designated surrogate includes the patient's diagnosis, prognosis, treatment options, and benefits and burdens of each option. Ideally, a surrogate named in an advance directive will have discussed the patient's wishes for medical and end-of-life care and be advised that he or she was a named surrogate. The surrogate can then use not only information in an advance directive (clear and convincing evidence) to make decisions, but also information provided during the discussions (substituted judgment). If none of this information is available, the surrogate(s) may need to use a best interest standard, weighing the benefits and burdens of the proposed interventions.

A surrogate's role is to make the same health care decisions that the patient would normally make. They do not, however, include decisions strictly within the professional realm, such as which antibiotic to use or how to perform a procedure. Surrogates should base their decisions about health care options on the best information they have about the patient. Optimally, they will know the patient well, be aware of his or her values, have discussed the patient's general health care wishes in advance, or have a written description of his or her wishes, such as the Physician Orders for Life-Sustaining Treatment (POLST) form. In that case, they may come close to adhering to the patient's preferences and values in decision-making, using what is often termed *substituted judgment.*

If this is not the case and there is inadequate evidence of the patient's preferences and values, the surrogate should base health care decisions on what most likely would promote the patient's well-being—usually described as using the *best interest standard.* Generally, the proxy must weigh the benefits (enough potential for improvement acceptable to the patient) and harms (including pain, risks, and potential impairment) to the patient of any intervention. A way for the proxy to objectify decisions rather than use his or her own values is to ask which option most reasonable persons would choose for themselves in similar circumstances.

In the case described, the physician would discuss the diagnosis, immediate plan (e.g., hospitalization, oxygen, and analgesia) and suggested referrals to the son. He can then decide on the course his mother will take and, of course, how much to tell her about the diagnosis.

Identifying a Surrogate (Health Care Proxy)

In this case, the patient, who retained decision-making capacity, verbally appointed her eldest son as her surrogate, despite the presence of her husband and several other adult children. More commonly, physicians identify surrogates for patients lacking decision-making capacity (temporarily or permanently) using advance directives or surrogate lists.

One of the most common types of advance directives is the durable power of attorney for health care. Its main function is to name potential health care surrogates for an individual. These advance directives often reside in the patient's health care record, since federal law (Federal Patient Self-Determination Act, effective December 1, 1991, OBRA-90; Pub.L. 101–508) requires that hospital patients (as well as those in nursing homes, home health agencies, hospices, and health maintenance organizations participating in the Medicare or Medicaid programs) be asked if they have an advance directive valid in their state and if they want to place a copy in their chart. In these documents, individuals can name any adult they choose as surrogate. Of course, if needed, the individual must be available and willing to serve as surrogate; individuals listed on these documents are often unavailable or unwilling to be a health care proxy. If a named proxy is available, he or she is the surrogate, no matter who else is available.

When no surrogate has been named, most hospital policies and many state statutes list the general hierarchy of people (if they are willing and available) to be the patient's surrogates. These are persons at least 18 years old who themselves have decision-making capacity. The most common list is the current spouse (not legally separated), parents, domestic partner, a majority of available siblings, close friend, attending physician—often in consultation with the institution's bioethics committee. (Domestic partner and close friend may be in different positions on the list, depending on the local laws and practices.) If none of these are available or willing to act as surrogate, or if there is disagreement among the same level of decision maker (i.e., siblings or parents), a court must intervene. This rarely occurs.

Special Cases: Guardians and Children

In the absence of a clear indication that the patient would, if competent, refuse the treatment, a surrogate decision maker must decide in the way that a reasonable person would in trying to achieve his own "best interest." In rare cases, patients have a court-appointed guardian for health care decisions. The guardian's decisions supersede those of both the patient and any other surrogates.

Parents are generally considered the surrogate decision makers for their minor, legally nonemancipated children. If parents appear not to be acting in their child's best interests, it requires legal intervention to change the decision maker.

The courts often act as the final adjudicators of disagreements over medical care. The courts, however, usually are neither expeditious nor necessarily cognizant of bioethical principles. They are instructed only to follow the societal values codified in the law. Many courts have suggested that whenever possible, health care decisions should remain at the bedside rather than in legal chambers.

BIOETHICS COMMITTEES AND CONSULTANTS

Multidisciplinary committees have been developed in most large hospitals to consult on cases with bioethical dilemmas and may also participate in surrogate decision-making. One of their functions is to consult prospectively and retrospectively on clinical cases and offer advice and conclusions to those directly involved, most often concerning the treatment or nontreatment of patients who lack decision-making capacity. Ethics committees usually do not act as the primary decision makers. Rather, the members serve as consultants, providing information, advising, and supporting the primary decision-making role of the patient-family-physician triad.

CASE RESOLUTION

This adult patient has decision-making capacity. Therefore, her right to make her own health care decisions, based on patient autonomy, must be respected. That includes naming her eldest son as her decision maker. This situation is very straightforward. The emergency physician needs no forms, policies, or consults to follow her oral directive.

KEY POINTS TO REMEMBER

- To make a health care decision, individuals (whether it be the patient or an adult surrogate) must have decision-making capacity.
- Based on patient autonomy (respect for persons), adults with decision-making capacity can make their own health care decisions, even if they contradict what their health care provider recommends.
- If a patient lacks decision-making capacity, his or her previously completed health care directive(s) take effect. These can be a living will, durable power of attorney for health care, POLST form, or a similar document.
- In a similar manner, if an adult patient wishes to orally designate another adult to make his or her health care decisions (as in this case), they may do that. These surrogates' decisions

carry the same weight as and replace any previously named surrogate.
- When no surrogate has been named, most hospital policies and many state statutes list the general hierarchy of people to be the patient's surrogates.

Suggested Reading

Abbott J. The POLST paradox: opportunities and challenges in honoring patient end-of-life wishes in the emergency department. *Ann Emerg Med*. 2018;*73*(3):294–301.

Iserson KV. A simplified prehospital advance directive law: Arizona's approach. *Ann Emerg Med*. 1993;*22*(11):1703–1710.

Iserson KV. Patient and surrogate autonomy: good idea—in theory. *Acad Emerg Med*. 2002;*9*(8):866.

Iserson KV. Principles of medical ethics. In: Marco C, Schears R (eds.), *Ethical dilemmas in emergency medicine*. New York: Cambridge University Press; 2015:1–17.

Iserson KV, Heine C. Bioethics. In: Walls RM, Hockberger RS, Gausche-Hill M, et al. (eds.), *Rosen's emergency medicine: concepts and clinical practice*, 9th edition. Philadelphia: Mosby; 2017: Chapter 10e.

Kraus CK, Marco CA. Shared decision making in the ED: ethical considerations. *Am J Emerg Med*. 2016 Aug 1;*34*(8):1668–1672.

7   Saving Grandpa?

Ahmed Shaikh and Jeremy R. Simon

An 85-year-old male with severe dementia is brought to the emergency department (ED) from his nursing home with fever and hypotension and found to have pneumonia. His blood pressure is 85/45 mm Hg, respiratory rate 32 breaths per minute, and oxygen saturation 93%. You realize that if the patient is not intubated, he will suffer respiratory failure and die in the ED. You not only tell this to the family, but also explain that you do not think you should intubate him because the patient will likely die in the intensive care unit (ICU) anyway, and that even if he does survive, he will likely need a tracheostomy and may have other complications of sepsis, such as amputations. The family nevertheless insists that you intubate him.

What do you do now?

FUTILE CARE

Medical providers frequently experience concern that they are offering what they suspect is futile care or feel frustrated that they are being asked to provide care that they believe is unwarranted. Another, more patient-focused, way to conceive of these cases is considering them to be care that is not beneficial to the patient. However, although the patient should always be our focus in medicine, the patient's perspective is not always the only relevant one in these discussions. Framing a discussion in terms of futility allows us to consider a wider range of issues. Either way, the concern is that there is no reason to provide the treatment in question. Such cases often result in significant distress for providers and calls to the ethics committee, and their resolution can be difficult. But before we consider how to respond to such dilemmas, we must first understand where they come from.

WHY IS FUTILITY AN ISSUE?

Futility first seems to have become a pressing issue for clinicians with the advent of a focus on patient autonomy in clinical decision-making. Before this, when physicians did what they thought best for the patient, there was little room for feeling pressed into treatments that seemed futile. If the physician thought it pointless, the treatment would not be undertaken. Once patients and their families became deeply involved in these decisions, physicians have found themselves in situations they would not have chosen.

A second factor was the development of powerful life support technologies, such as ventilators and extracorporeal membrane oxygenation (ECMO). Suddenly, there were many patients being kept alive for significant lengths of time in situations that, at least to some, appeared pointless and hopeless. Physicians often find these cases difficult to deal with and view the hopelessness of the case as demonstrating the futility of the care.

WHAT IS FUTILE CARE?

But, what do we mean by "futile" here in the first place? The *Random House Dictionary* defines *futile* as "incapable of producing a result; ineffective, useless." However, it is extraordinarily rare that a treatment we are considering cannot produce any result. Compressions on an elderly patient with met-astatic disease *will* circulate blood. Intubating a patient who will die soon regardless *will* ventilate and oxygenate the patient. This disconnect between the dictionary definition of futility and the types of cases physicians refer to as futile has led to several different proposals for a definition of futility in the medical context.

Schneiderman, Jecker, and Jonsen (1990) identified two kinds of futility: quantitative and qualitative. *Quantitative* futility refers to treatments that have an extremely low likelihood of success. *Qualitative* futility refers to treatments that preserve life but leave the patient completely dependent on intensive care or permanently unconscious. Brody and Halevy (1995) defined four types of futility. *Physiologic* futility refers to treatment that, like defibrillation for asystole, simply cannot yield the desired physiological effect. *Imminent demise* futility refers to efforts that may accomplish their narrow purpose but will not change the fact that the patient will die very soon anyway, such as cardiac compressions on a patient with metastatic cancer. *Lethal condition* futility refers to cases where the patient will live somewhat longer than in the last case, but will die soon of their underlying condition. An example of this might be cardiac compressions in an end-stage liver disease patient who is not eligible for a transplant and has only weeks to months to live. Finally, *qualitative* futility refers to treatment that will leave the patient with an unacceptable quality of life, without defining what is unacceptable. Others see futility as referring not to a specific class of treatments but as "the end of a spectrum of low-efficacy therapies," while still others argue that futility is different from low efficacy.

These and other conflicting accounts of futility can make it difficult to decide which treatments count as futile, let alone what to do in such cases. As we shall see, both of these problems can be addressed by approaching the matter from a different perspective. Before we get there, though, we must consider the clinical and legal environment in which we work.

THE EMERGENCY DEPARTMENT

The spectrum of futility decisions in the ED is proportional to the seem-ingly infinite spectrum of clinical scenarios faced by emergency physicians. A resuscitation attempt may be prolonged, possibly long after it seems it should have stopped, or an open thoracostomy attempted in blunt trauma despite evidence that it is useless. Finally, some cases may appear futile even when the treatment "works," as in the successful return of spontaneous circulation to a patient whose downtime was long enough that the patient will undoubtedly suffer profound neurological damage.

Another set of cases that may raise futility concerns in the ED are those where the treatment itself will work, but does not seem worth doing. Should one intubate a patient for respiratory failure if that patient had previously expressed a desire not to undergo prolonged intubation and one believes that will be the outcome? Should one spend time aggressively stabilizing a patient with a ruptured abdominal aortic aneurysm if that patient will expire soon after arrival in the ICU because he is not a surgical candidate? Should one treat a severely demented patient in septic shock, with its attendant risk of loss of limbs and so on?

In addition to unique clinical situations, the practice environment of the ED creates challenges to resolving these cases. As we shall see, communication is key to their resolution. The ED presents many barriers to effective communication. First, there is little time in which to develop the trust and understanding that is key in successful doctor-patient relationships. There also is scant opportunity to explore patient goals and desires. Finally, even when some of these problems are overcome, many decisions must be made urgently, with little time to discuss them.

LEGAL CONSIDERATIONS

In addition to understanding the clinical environment, it is important to understand the legal milieu as well. If one is thinking about futility, one is thinking about withdrawing or withholding care, and such situations can have legal implications. The first is malpractice. A family that believes something appropriate was not done for a loved one may sue. State laws may also be relevant. Some states, such as Texas, have legally mandated processes for physicians to follow when considering withholding or withdrawing treatment. Others limit the situations in which a physician may have the potential make such a decision. In New York, for instance, physicians cannot declare care to be futile over a surrogate's objection without judicial review. Being aware of the legal ramifications of decisions is always important.

BEYOND FUTILITY: COMMUNICATION AND HUMILITY

How then can we best respond to situations in which we feel we are being asked to render inappropriate or useless treatment? The first step is to prepare for, and potentially avoid, such conflicts by building rapport with the patient and family before such a point is reached. As we noted, this can be difficult in the ED, but it can be done. Sit and pay attention when talking with the patient and family. Attend to the patient's comfort when possible with an extra sheet or a cup of water. Speak clearly and without jargon or advanced vocabulary. All of these can help build trust.

Sometimes, however, even the most well-meaning physicians and family members (and it is usually family members involved in these sorts of cases, not patients) can disagree about what is appropriate. In such a case, the next steps depend on the immediacy of the situation.

If the decision does not need to be made at that moment, one should ask whether it needs to be made in the ED at all. If not, then it probably should not be. Highly charged decisions such as withholding care should be made in the calmest environment possible. Even the ICU is calmer than the ED.

If the decision cannot be deferred, the first step should not be deciding whether the treatment would be futile. It should be engaging in more communication. Does the family understand why you do not want to do what they are asking? Perhaps they do not realize how invasive or inappropriate their request is, like defibrillation for asystole. Do you understand why the family is requesting what they are? Perhaps they will tell you how the patient had consistently chosen even painful and invasive treatments that most people would refuse, if there was any chance that they might help. Or perhaps they understand that the intervention in question will at most only delay death by a few hours, but they want time for other family to gather. In these situations, treatments that originally seemed futile may come to appear appropriate.

Also important is gathering more information if possible. Are there others who know more about the patient's expressed wishes, or are there advanced directives or Medical Orders for Life-Sustaining Treatment (MOLST)/ Physician Orders for Life-Sustaining Treatment (POLST) forms that have not yet been considered? Any of these sources could shed important light on the patient's wishes and help resolve a conflict.

If disagreement persists, one can bring in others who have not yet been involved in the discussion, such as other family members, friends, clergy, private physicians or ethics consultants. The new perspective of these additions, who also may be less emotionally involved in the case, may help break the impasse.

When an impasse persists despite all attempts at resolution, which will hopefully be a rare occurrence, or when the decision must be made emergently and there is no time for all of the actions mentioned, the emergency physician must decide how to proceed clinically. In making such decisions, the physician must act carefully and with humility, with a bias toward continuing treatment. There are many reasons for this. First, irreversible decisions, which many decisions to withhold or withdraw treatment are, must be made with the utmost confidence, which rarely can be achieved in the ED. Second, many times when one says that treatment is futile, or nonbeneficial, what one means is the life that the patient will be left with after the treatment is not worthwhile, either because it will be too short or because it will be too disabled. However, while physicians are experts in medicine, they are not experts in meaningful lives. What is meaningful is for each person (perhaps speaking through surrogates) to decide for themselves. If a physician is thinking of stopping care in the ED for these reasons, he or she is likely out of bounds.

There is one set of circumstances in which an emergency physician would be justified in withholding therapy, even over the objections of family. Physicians are under no obligation to supply treatments that are simply ineffective in a given case, such as defibrillation for asystole or thoracotomy for blunt trauma. In such a case, they may follow the American College of Emergency Physicians' (2017) "Non-Beneficial ('Futile') Emergency Medical Interventions Policy," which states that "[p]hysicians are under no ethical obligation to render treatments that they judge have no realistic likelihood of medical benefit to the patient."

It is important that whenever care is withheld over objections that the reasons for doing so are explained clearly, calmly, and sympathetically to the family and friends involved, and that the actual withdrawal or withholding be done in a compassionate manner. It may also be appropriate to notify hospital risk management of any such decision before it is acted on.

CASE RESOLUTION

The family of our patient was asking that you intubate him even though you thought that not doing so was in the patient's best interests. The family then explains to you that they consider every moment of life precious and, furthermore, that there are several more children and grandchildren who would want to come from out of town before the patient dies. With this understanding, you are able to intubate the patient without misgivings. You also realize that even without these factors, it would be inappropriate to withhold intubation if the family judged intubation to be appropriate.

KEY POINTS TO REMEMBER

- Futility, or nonbeneficial treatment, is a difficult concept to define and ought to be used with caution, if at all.
- There can be legal ramifications, or limitations, on unilateral decision-making by physicians.
- Communication is key to avoiding conflicts over whether a given treatment ought to be undertaken.
- One should be hesitant to declare any treatment in the ED to be futile.
- In those limited cases in which it is appropriate, where the treatment is truly useless under the circumstances, be sure to act with kindness and compassion to the patient and his or her loved ones when delivering and acting on the decision.

Suggested Reading

American College of Emergency Physicians Clinical Policy: Nonbeneficial ("Futile") Emergency Medical Interventions. (Revised January 2017). Reaffirmed October 2008, October 2002. Originally approved March 1998, https://www.acep.org/patient-care/policy-statements/nonbeneficial-futile-emergency-medical-interventions/. Accessed February 1, 2020.

Brody BA, Halevy A. Is futility a futile concept? *J Med Philos.* 1995;*20*:123–144.

Helft PR, Siegler M, Lantos J. The rise and fall of the futility movement. *N Engl J Med.* 2000;*343*(4):293–296.

Marco CA, Larkin GL. Ethics seminars: case studies in "futility" —challenges for academic emergency medicine. *Acad Emerg Med.* 2000;*7*(10):1147–1151.

Marco CA, Larkin GL, Moskop JC, Derse AR. Determinations of futility in emergency medicine. *Ann Emerg Med.* 2000;*35*(6):604–612.

O'Connor AE, Winch S, Lukin W, Parker M. Emergency medicine and futile care: taking the road less travelled. *Emerg Med Australas.* 2011;*23*(5):640–643.

Pope TM. Legal briefing: futile or non-beneficial treatment. *J Clin Ethics.* 2011;*22*(3):277–296.

Pope TM. Dispute resolution mechanisms for intractable medical futility disputes. *N Y Law School Law Rev.* 2014;*58*:347–368.

Schneiderman LJ, Jecker NS, Jonsen AR. Medical futility: its meaning and ethical implications. *Ann Int Med.* 1990;*112*(12):949–954.

Simon JR, Krauss C, Rosenberg M, Wang DH, Clayborne EP, Derse AR. "Futile care" — an emergency medicine approach: ethical and legal considerations. *Ann Emerg Med.* 2017;*70*(5):707–713.

8 Failed Suicide Attempt in the Terminally Ill

Kenneth V. Iserson and Eileen F. Baker

Emergency medical services (EMS) brings a 46-year-old man to the emergency department (ED) for a medication overdose. The patient's wife called when he appeared to be in respiratory distress. He has a long history of multiple sclerosis (MS), with recent, rapid progression of symptoms. His wife explains that he was losing his ability to grasp objects and feed himself. The patient has had episodes of hypoxia, sleep apnea, and respiratory difficulty. His doctor was considering tracheostomy.

On arrival, the patient was intubated by the paramedics. He has sluggish pupils, and deep tendon reflexes are absent, without posturing. His wife admits that he had been hoarding his opioids and benzodiazepines in preparation for ending his life. You suspect that the patient could not have taken the overdose without help, and you believe his wife gave him the medications. She shows you his advance directive, which indicates he did not wish to be resuscitated. She insists that he be extubated and reminds you that he named her as his medical decision maker.

What do you do now?

PHYSICIAN-ASSISTED SUICIDE AND ACTS OF SELF-HARM

Physician-assisted suicide (PAS), also known as physician-assisted death (PAD) or physician aid-in-dying, denotes the practice of physicians prescribing medications to terminally ill patients, at their request. The patients can later elect to take these medications to hasten their death. This is an explicit arrangement between patient and their physician, although physicians are not present when the medications are taken. There is no role for emergency physicians (EPs) in this process—unless something goes wrong.

While PAS is legal in only a few states, all 50 states have statutes upholding competent patients' autonomy to make choices regarding end-of-life care, including limitations of resuscitative efforts. Statutes permit PAS in Colorado; Washington, DC; Hawaii; Oregon; Vermont; New Jersey, Maine, and Washington State (CNN Library, 2019). Court rulings permit it in Montana, and California. While the statutory language varies, they generally require a physician licensed in the state where the patient resides to prescribe such medication. Patients must have a terminal illness with a prognosis of 6 months or less to live. (Of course, such prognoses can err enormously.) These laws protect physicians from prosecution for prescribing medications to hasten a patient's death.

While EPs are unlikely to be involved in prescribing medications for PAS, they may be involved in the care of patients who experience problems with a suicide attempt after choosing PAS. As in this case example, in states where PAS is not legal, terminal patients often use hoarded medications or other means to end their lives. Traditionally, and consistent with professional and societal expectations, EPs aggressively treat patients presenting after attempting suicide. This includes supporting adverse medication effects, treating injuries, obtaining a psychiatric evaluation, and admitting the patient to the hospital (with or without patient consent) if indicated.

The clinical rationale for resuscitating the patient after a failed suicide attempt is based on the idea that those who attempt suicide are performing an irrational act. The patient is assumed to be suffering from a mental illness that impairs judgment. Once the patient's condition is stabilized, it is hoped that the patient's underlying mental illness can be addressed, and that the individual no longer will wish to commit suicide.

However, the analogy between those who attempt suicide through PAS and other patients who attempt suicide is incongruent. Advocates of PAS argue that those who opt for PAS are not arriving at this choice as the result of severe mental disease, but rather through careful consideration of the wish to avoid the suffering and debility accompanying terminal illness. They state that in those with painful, progressive terminal illnesses, the goal to protect the patient from harm may not be to prolong life, but rather to hasten death. Proponents assert that a prescription for a lethal dose of medication is arrived at through careful discussions with the patient and an assessment of the patient's medical condition, mental capacity, and expressed wishes.

A more apt analogy for those who attempt suicide through PAS is to terminally ill patients with advance directives who indicate their desire to forgo life-prolonging treatment and who arrive in the ED seeking palliative care for pain or other intolerable symptoms. Treating terminally ill patients in the ED is not uncommon. Families often panic when seeing a loved one in the process of dying, even if provided medications to ease suffering, as in hospice situations. At times, the patient may appear to require more care than the family can manage or need additional or alternative medications to allow the patient to be comfortable. Discovering a loved one after a failed suicide attempt is another, albeit less common, reason for presentation, usually via EMS, to the ED.

The question is whether the patient with a terminal condition who attempted suicide in this case is similar in a morally relevant way to patients with a PAS. This already poses something of a legal and ethical quandary because PAS provides statutory permission to end one's life that is absent in other suicide attempts.

Some suggest that if there is doubt about the patient's condition and wishes, the EP should sustain life until further information is available to fully appreciate the patient's condition and wishes. At issue is the concern that a decision to withhold or withdraw life-sustaining treatment usually is irreversible. But if we accept that the patient in this case indeed is seeking palliative care, EPs should respect the patient's right to refuse unwanted treatment by means of an advance directive or at the direction of a health care agent. In this case, it would be acting in accord with the request of the patient's wife. This fulfills the moral duty of EPs to honor the wishes of a terminally ill patient by refraining from resuscitative efforts. Conversely, as discussed in material that follows, the EP, who has not signed on to participate, may have moral or professional objections to participating in this process.

ETHICAL CONSIDERATIONS

In cases such as this, EPs cannot know the patient's mental state or whether it was an autonomous rational decision when he or she attempted suicide. While family and medical decision makers such as a health care power of attorney may disagree with the wishes of the patient, ideally the wishes of family members should not override a patient's autonomous choice. It is also important to note that patients may choose to change their mind about end-of-life wishes at any time. Nevertheless, respect for autonomy is not absolute. EPs have a duty to protect patients from harm. The decision to override a patient's choices expressed in an advance directive calls on ED staff to act under the principles of beneficence and nonmaleficence. This presumes that it would be more beneficial to preserve and extend the patient's life than to allow him or her to die, or that at the very least, the EP should "do no harm" in passively permitting the patient's death.

Even in states where PAS is legal, EPs may not be supportive of such statutes. While the patient's physician may have voluntarily agreed to participate in the PAS process, EPs are involuntarily drawn into it if the suicide attempt fails. They then have three options: to actively assist the patient's dying (active euthanasia), permit the patient to die without active interventions (passive euthanasia—a misleading term, but that's what we have), and actively intervene trying to prevent death.

The first option, actively assisting the patient to complete suicide (active euthanasia) honors the patient's wishes but places the physician in legal peril. No US jurisdictions allow this. Further, EPs generally lack the long-term relationship with their patients that is required to become knowledgeable about the patient's condition, prognosis, capacity, and values. Even in states where PAS is legal, physicians who choose to assist suicide face ethical criticism from colleagues and risk public perception of the hospital as a place where patients are killed intentionally and involuntarily.

The second option, permitting the patient to die without active interventions (passive euthanasia) while providing palliative care has the moral advantage of honoring the patient's desire to forgo life-prolonging care and avoiding additional suffering from the terminal disease or from resuscitative efforts. This also may allow time to gather reliable evidence about the patient's condition and end-of-life wishes. However, in the absence of adequate information, such measures may allow a patient to die who desires treatment and life-prolonging measures. Additionally, it fails to honor the request of someone who has attempted to end his or her life, who seeks assistance in carrying out the suicidal intent.

The third option follows standard ED practice. Laws vary across states, but most institutional policies allow practitioners to withdraw from providing care in a situation that violates their convictions, provided an alternative professional is willing to assume responsibility for the patient. Life-sustaining treatment can be withdrawn at a later time. One rationale is that intervening to preserve the patient's life after a failed suicide attempt may afford the treatment team to buy time until more information is available about the patient's wishes. But when reliable information about the patient's wishes is clear, preserving life may prolong the unwanted suffering and indignity of terminal illness that the patient was trying to avoid. However, this simply passes the ultimate decision on to the inpatient physician.

CASE RESOLUTION

In the case provided, you suspect that the patient could not have self-administered his overdose. What is your legal obligation in this case? This is a situation the EP should not face alone. Consultation with the hospital's ethics committee, hospital attorney, or risk management department should be attempted in real time. Undoubtedly, there are situations in which the patient's spouse acts compassionately in assisting her husband to commit suicide. But placing one's self in the situation of deciding whether the actions are illegal, and whether the wife should be reported to authorities, is not the purview of the physician. Giving medication to complete the suicide places the EP at both legal and moral peril. When the patient's wishes are clear, as in this case, offering palliative treatment provides care in keeping with the patient's desire to avoid pain and suffering. In situations in which questions exist regarding the patient's wishes, a more conservative approach, aimed at stabilizing the patient, should be sought. Clarification of the patient's medical condition, end-of-life wishes, and health care proxy may be established, with care to continue once those wishes are established.

You examine the advance directive the patient's wife provides, designating her as his health care proxy. Review of the medical record reveals a long relationship with a local primary care provider. You contact the primary care physician and explain the situation. She empathizes with the patient, his wife, and the situation in which you find yourself. She confirms that the patient had discussed his wish for palliative care and notes that while the patient had mild bouts of depression, he was clear and consistent in expression of his desire to avoid prolonged suffering. You contact the hospitalist and explain the situation. You agree that the patient will be extubated and maintained on supplemental oxygen, while awaiting placement on the hospital floor under do not resuscitate (DNR) orders. A palliative care consultation also is arranged to manage the patient's respiratory distress and optimize his comfort. The patient dies within 12 hours, with his wife at his bedside.

KEY POINTS TO REMEMBER

- While PAS only is legalized in a few states, all states have provisions for upholding the autonomy of competent patients to make decisions about end-of-life care.
- Emergency Physicians are unlikely to prescribe medications for PAS but may be asked to care for those seeking palliative care at the end of life or who have a failed suicide attempt.
- The clinical rationale for resuscitating the patient after a failed suicide attempt is based on the idea that those who attempt suicide are performing an irrational act. However, the analogy between those who attempt suicide through PAS and other patients who attempt suicide is incongruent because patients seeking PAS have had time for careful consideration of treatment options and have undergone a thorough assessment

of their medical condition, mental capacity, and expressed wishes.
- Three options are available to the EP caring for a terminally ill patient with a failed suicide attempt: to assist a patient in completing an intended suicide (active euthanasia), to offer palliative care only (passive euthanasia), or to override the patient's wishes and provide life-saving treatment (standard treatment).
- Assisting in suicide (active euthanasia) is not legal anywhere in the United States.
- Consultation with the hospital's ethics committee, legal counsel, or risk management department is advisable.
- When the patient's wishes are clear, offering palliative treatment provides care in keeping with the patient's desire to avoid pain and suffering.
- In situations in which questions exist regarding the patient's wishes, a more conservative approach, aimed at stabilizing the patient, should be sought.

Suggested Reading

American College of Emergency Medicine. Policy statement: ethical issues at the end of life Approved April 2014. https://www.acep.org/patient-care/policy-statements/ethical-issues-at-the-end-of-life/. Accessed March 24, 2019.

American Medical Association. Chapter 5: Opinions on caring for patients at the end of life. https://www.ama-assn.org/sites/ama-assn.org/files/corp/media-browser/code-of-medical-ethics-chapter-5.pdf. Accessed March 24, 2019.

Geppert, C. Saving life or respecting autonomy: the ethical dilemma of DNR orders in patients who attempt suicide. *Internet J Law, Healthcare Ethics*. 2010;7(1).

Moskop, JC, Iserson, KV. Emergency physicians and physician-assisted suicide, part II: emergency care for patients who have attempted physician-assisted suicide. *Ann Emerg Med*. 2001 November;38(5):576–582.

CNN Library. Physician-assisted suicide fast facts. Updated 9:16 AM ET, Thursday August 1, 2019, https://www.ama-assn.org/sites/ama-assn.org/files/corp/media-browser/code-of-medical-ethics-chapter-5.pdf. Accessed February 1, 2020.

Willful death and painful decisions: a failed assisted suicide. *Camb Q Healthc Ethics*. 1992;1(2):147–158.

9 The Doctor's Dilemma

Raquel M. Schears and
Markayle R. Schears

A 65-year-old farmer is brought into the emergency department (ED) by helicopter from the scene. The patient sustained a self-inflicted shotgun injury to the face a half hour earlier and had yelled for help, alerting his wife, who called 911. They noted the patient was conversant and refusing transport or intervention. He consented to blow-by oxygen and intravenous (IV) placement and required continuous suctioning to manage the blood loss from his facial wounds. His wife produced a typed do not resuscitate/intubate (DNR/I) document signed by his doctor the day before, as earlier in the week her husband was diagnosed based on a liver biopsy with terminal cancer. He refused to undergo chemotherapy, and the liver tumor was inoperable. On arrival, he had a Glasgow Coma Scale (GCS) score of 15, heart rate of 108 beats per minute, blood pressure of 122/78 mm Hg, and respiratory rate of 22 breaths per minute with O_2 saturations in the high 90s. Examination was only notable for massive midface trauma with no discernible maxilla, nose, or eyes. The mandible was intact, but there was concern for blood, bone, and tooth fragments threatening airway patency.

What do you do now?

PHYSICIAN-UNASSISTED SUICIDE

Suicidal ideation and attempted suicide are important presenting complaints in the ED. The juxtaposition of self-inflicted gunshot wounds and self-reported no code status may serve to amplify the moral distress of medical decision-making for emergency providers. That the apparent suicide involves a terminal patient, whose diagnosis portends a relentless, progressive course, requires investigation. It is reasonable for the trauma team to obtain the input of hospital legal counsel and a clinical ethics consultation to sort out difficult scenarios before and after the clinical encounter. Certainly, involving more clinical resources and hospital expertise to navigate the complex issues of this case is the first thing one should do, possibly even before the patient arrives.

Suicide-related ED visits have become increasingly common over the last 20 years, and suicide is recognized as a major public health concern. More Americans die annually from suicide than traffic accidents, HIV/AIDS, and homicides combined. Suicide remains the 10th leading cause of death overall in the United States. Numerous cases in the literature have been reported of patients who attempted suicide and presented to the ED with an advance directive (AD) stating that they do not want resuscitation. Physicians may feel conflicted in these situations, trying to reconcile their initial instinct to resuscitate, and their professional responsibility to intervene with a suicidal patient, with the legal mandate to respect a patient's expressed wishes. Further complicating these situations is the professional debate ongoing in the United States regarding the acceptability of physician-assisted suicide. Currently, 10 states (Oregon, Washington, Vermont, Maine, New Jersey, Colorado, Washington DC, California, Montana, and Hawaii) allow physician-assisted suicide (CNN Library, 2019).

From a hospital legal perspective, the advice offered is typically confirmatory of the physicians' clinical impulses to resuscitate first and ask questions later when confronted with life-threatening emergencies. The emergency exception to informed consent is generally cited for this approach. Yet, there are circumstances when the exemption thresholds for an emergency are crossed but a patient has left clear directions that they would not want treatment. A decision to proceed with resuscitation should not be based solely on the urgency of the medical condition; it must also consider whether an AD is present, and, if so, if it is a valid AD that represents an enduring wish.

Emergency medical services (EMS), in the case at hand, had contacted Medical Control (MC) in the ED and acted in support of the autonomy of the patient to refuse intubation. They felt that the airway could be temporized in transport, as had been done at the scene. Also, the paramedics were not confident they could intubate due to the shattered midface. Given that the patient was oriented and interactive, practitioners were concerned that they could face assault or battery charges related to unconsented intubation. The paramedics discounted the MC assertion that the DNR/I status be considered invalid due to the suicide attempt. Fortunately, the patient maintained his airway during the flight with oxygen saturations holding in the upper 90s. On arrival in the ED, the existence of his AD became a moot point because the patient was still conversant and responsive. Assessing the patient's injury and respecting his words with cooperative medical actions remained the first duty of the physicians.

From an ethical standpoint, having a crucial conversation with the patient to ensure "the needs of the patient come first" is a priority and supports autonomous decision-making during the clinical care episode. In the moment, people may change their minds, and they may request rescue as they are frightened and vulnerable. This patient was gurgling blood and struggling to breathe. Such actions do not necessarily mean that one revokes one's AD. One may want to be saved from immediate symptoms (air hunger and pain) but still hold the overriding wish not to be kept alive.

As this case demonstrates, whether an AD is valid does not hinge on the lethality of the means used in the suicidal presentation. Rather, the directive only comes into force when the person is incapable of communicating his wishes. In most situations, an AD matches what our clinical judgment would support (i.e., incapacitated terminally ill patients who refuse life-sustaining treatments) or we are able to verify the wishes with a substitute decision maker and we must honor these. When a patient who has attempted suicide presents with an AD there are many reasons why we should question the validity of these documents in the ED and treat the acute medical issues.

On arrival in the trauma bay, this patient was immediately assessed by the physician in charge. She informed him that she was concerned he wouldn't be able to breathe on his own much longer because of the significant facial trauma. She asked him if he would like a "tube in his throat also known as intubation" so he wouldn't be breathing on his own. He said "yes," indicating he did want this. He surprised the doctor with his response, so she paused the activity in the room and repeated her question to the patient who again replied in the affirmative, that he wanted to be intubated. There was general agreement he had requested intubation and the physician carried out the procedure successfully.

Intubating him when he requested it was appropriate. The due diligence the EMS providers took not to pursue further intervention when he refused intubation earlier on the scene was also appropriate. This preserved the patient's autonomy and bought time to sort out his wishes while managing his symptoms cooperatively. Subsequently, head computed tomography (Figure 9.1) was obtained and confirmed extensive facial trauma. He was taken to the operating room and prepped for surgery, awaiting the arrival

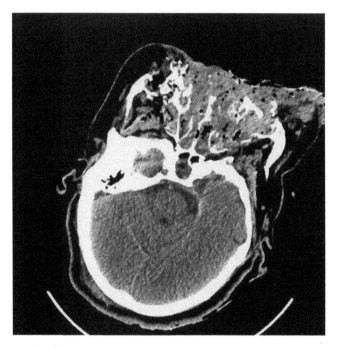

FIGURE 9.1 Head CT with maxillofacial cut. Shattered midface, frontal subarachnoid hemorrhage, intracranial shrapnel, and pneumocephalus.

of his wife and health care power of attorney to obtain consent for the operation.

Invoking an ethics consult early on turned out to be a good call in hindsight. In conversation with the patient's wife, it became clear his desire to forgo treatment was consistent over time; he refused chemotherapy for the cancer and wanted to avoid a protracted death. With the help of the Ethics Consultation Service, the decision was made to abort the surgical plan and support end of life with medical management and withdrawal of care in the surgical intensive care unit. The patient was extubated and died peacefully shortly thereafter. Clergy provided support for the patient and his wife during the hospital stay, and grief counselors were active in helping the wife in the outpatient setting.

The larger unresolved ethical issue of this case is the fact of his suicide attempt. Emergency physicians are unaccustomed to standing by as someone dies from suicide. Practitioners assume that mental illness drives the decision to commit suicide, and ignore patients' pleas to allow them to die. The question is, if a patient overdoses, for example, and a family member comes in with an AD that says "no extraordinary measures" should we actually respect it?

A second consideration in the general context of an apparent suicide arises. Does the fact that a patient has attempted suicide alter our legal and professional responsibilities regarding ADs? Every jurisdiction in North America has legislation that allows emergency physicians to hold suicidal patients until they can be further assessed by a psychiatrist. Acutely suicidal patients often have a mental health condition that impairs their capacity to make treatment decisions. Suicidal ideation is typically transient, and many of the underlying conditions that contribute to its development are treatable. ADs are intended to convey enduring wishes that represent the patient's core values. It is the very rare circumstance (albeit this case) where a suicide attempt would meet these criteria, and it would be extremely difficult to verify this in the ED context. For this reason, emergency physicians generally should treat suicidal patients despite an AD to the contrary. Another exception to the rule may exist for physicians in states where physician-assisted suicide is legal. Patients in these jurisdictions who have attempted suicide as part of a legal and professionally sanctioned process may not die outside the hospital as expected. Family or friends may call 911, and the patient arrives in the ED. It is imperative the patient present clear and assessable documentation establishing that they meet predetermined criteria for medical assistance in dying. The emergency physician must be able to establish this was a legal act that occurred only after appropriate assessment of the patient, both to ensure vulnerable patients are not denied appropriate care, and to protect emergency physicians against a legal action or professional complaint.

CASE RESOLUTION

What was different in this case? One exceptional consideration in apparent suicide presentations is whether treatment can be effective. In this case, and in others involving, for example, ingestion of large quantities of medication or severe trauma, there is a very low likelihood that any intervention could produce a good outcome. In these cases, the basis for withholding treatment is not the AD, but the likelihood that the treatment wouldn't succeed.

Nevertheless, emergency physicians may struggle with the tension between beneficence and respecting patient autonomy, when normally we would assume that someone committing suicide had questionable decision-making capacity. In our 65-year-old gentleman with terminal liver cancer, a DNR order, and a self-inflicted gunshot wound to the head, facial reconstruction or even facial transplantation has a very low likelihood of producing a good outcome. Recovery would be a difficult road, so it is possible to empathize with the patient's desire to forgo further treatment.

Alternatively, had the capacitated patient with a terminal diagnosis and botched suicide attempt not consented to intubation, upholding his wishes for rational suicide and nonintervention might have been a far harder pill for the physicians to swallow. Suspending our instinct to intervene with life sustaining treatment from the ED is difficult. Even when death is believed to be the lesser evil by a terminal patient acting in the extreme, physicians rarely acknowledge there are fates worse than death. This case also introduces the concern of whether death can legitimately be controlled as a benefit to such patients. Assisted suicide has a narrow definition that doesn't directly apply to ED practice in most states. Suffice it to say, when 'the needs of the patient come first," physicians must be prepared, in exceptional circumstances, to step back and allow death to occur. Respecting the right of patients to refuse care, the very skill at which we excel as clinicians, is a true test of professional fiber.

KEY POINTS TO REMEMBER

- The urgency of the need for treatment is not justification to override valid refusals or deny requests from patients with ADs.
- Patients with decisional capacity have the right to refuse life-sustaining treatments if their refusal represents an informed decision and enduring wish.
- There is a strong legal and professional justification for holding suicidal patients for psychiatric assessment, and treating their emergent medical concerns *first*, even if there is a valid AD that asks that treatment be withheld. While some states allow physician-assisted suicide, the conditions that must be met are generally not verifiable in the emergency setting.
- In cases where a patient who has attempted suicide presents with an AD refusing treatment, the emergency physician should recognize their mandate to hold and treat emergency conditions in suicidal patients, and evaluate whether it is one of the exceptional circumstances where an AD may be valid. The physician should also consider if their proposed treatment can have the desired effect.

Suggested Reading

Barber, CW, Miller, MJ. Reducing a suicidal person's access to lethal means of suicide: a research agenda. *Am J Prev Med.* 2014;*47*:S264–S272.

Butkus R, Doherty R, Bornstein SS. Health and Public Policy Committee of the American College of Physicians. Reducing firearm injuries and deaths in the United States: a position paper from the American College of Physicians. *Ann Intern Med.* 2018;*69*:704–707.

CNN Library. Physician-Assisted Suicide Fast Facts. Updated 9:16 AM ET, Thursday August 1, 2019, https://www.ama-assn.org/sites/ama-assn.org/files/corp/media-browser/code-of-medical-ethics-chapter-5.pdf. Accessed February 1, 2020.

David AS, Hotopf M, Moran P, et al. Mentally disordered or lacking capacity? Lessons for managing serious deliberate self harm. *Br Med J.* 2010;*341*:587–589.

Dresser R. Suicide attempts and treatment refusals. *Hastings Center Report.* 2010;*40*:10–11.

Krysinska K, Lester D, Martin G. Suicide behavior after a traumatic event. *J Trauma Nursing.* 2009;*16*:103–110.

Olfson M, Marcus SC, Bridge JA. Focusing suicide prevention on periods of high risk. *JAMA.* 2014;*311*:1107–1108.

Olick RS. Defining features of advance directives in law and clinical practice. *Chest.* 2012;*141*:232–238.

Palmer RB, Iserson KV. The critical patient who refuses treatment: an ethical dilemma. *J Emerg Med.* 1997;15:729–733.

Pauls M, Larkin GL, Schears RM. Advance directives and suicide attempts-ethical considerations in light of Carter v. Canada, SCC 5. *Canadian Journal of Emerg Med.* 2015;*17*:562–564.

VanderWeele TJ, Li S, Tsai AC, et al. Association between religious service attendance and lower suicide rates among US women. *JAMA Psychiatry.* 2016;*73*:845–851.

Woolley SJ. Jehovah's Witnesses in the emergency department: what are their rights? *J Emerg Med.* 2005;*22*:869–871.

10 Hide and Seek

Purva Grover

You walk into a patient room for which the chief complaint
on the tracking board says, "ingestion." The patient is
19 years old and tried to hurt herself by consuming a handful
of ibuprofen pills. Her mother is surprised and just can't
wrap her head around the "why." The patient tells you in
confidence that her father has been touching her private
parts for many years, and she wants to die but does NOT
want to report this.

What do you do now?

MANDATORY REPORTING

Incidences of child abuse and neglect have a profound effect on the lives of many children across the United States. Therefore, all states have set in place variations of mandatory reporting laws in order to decrease and prevent these incidents from occurring. These laws help ensure that cases of child abuse are reported to the proper authorities. Mandatory reporting laws differ for each state when it comes to child abuse, which includes physical abuse, sexual abuse, and emotional abuse. However, it's important to remember that many of these laws also cover child neglect. In some states, these laws require that people in certain professions report child abuse and neglect to a proper authority, such as a law enforcement agency or child protective services. In other states, the mandatory reporting laws require *any* person who suspects child abuse or neglect report any such instance. According to information provided to the US Department of Human and Health Services (HHS), 48 states have mandatory reporting laws requiring certain people to report child abuse and neglect. These individuals usually are people who have frequent contact with children because of their occupation.

Situations in which mandatory reporters must inform authorities vary depending on state mandatory reporting laws. However, according to the HHS, there are typically two standards regarding when a report should be made:

- When the reporter has reason to believe or suspect that a child has been abused or neglected.
- When the reporter sees a child being subjected to harm or knows of conditions that would reasonably result in harm to the child.

A major cause of physician underreporting is the fact that the abused patient tends not to have a presenting complaint that is a type of abuse. Rather, the presenting complaint may be unexplained genitourinary injury, undue parental anxiety focused on the genitourinary system, prepubertal venereal disease, teenage pregnancy, or nonspecific behavioral problems. The antithesis, of course, is the case in which parents fear a sexual assault has occurred and, therefore, present the child for evaluation. There may be no verification of any such incident by history or physical examination, yet the patient is recorded as a case of alleged sexual assault. Physical injury is involved in a relatively small proportion of alleged sexual assault cases seen by physicians. The incidence of positive physical findings has been reported to range from 10% to 50%. But important, too, is the fact that delays in seeking medical corroboration of the assault interfere with the possibility of noting positive physical findings, as does washing the child prior to taking the child to the hospital.

The families of sexually abused children play a major role in deciding whether an incident is reported and in determining the delay. Perhaps the child does not confide in anyone or, if questioned, denies anything happened. When informed, a family member may judge the accuracy of the confession and decide either not to act on it or to delay any action in exchange for time to ponder the next move.

Again, the type of sexual abuse may be the deciding factor. In the case of incest, the abuser probably is the economic or emotional head of the household. Pressing charges could provoke physical abuse and would also lead to public disclosure of a very serious offense that is likely to compromise family status. Many of these same feelings and attitudes also are present when the assailant is an acquaintance. If the assailant is a stranger, the family may be most concerned about the possibility of rebuke from the community. The child who is abused may be too fearful of physical harm and social rejection to want a problem made known. Such a child feels fear, guilt, parental rejection, and anxiety about family disintegration. Studies exemplify the one aspect of this reporting problem that remains constant: the assumption that whatever figures are reported, they surely are not complete.

ETHICAL CONSIDERATIONS

The overall management of sexual abuse must be multidisciplinary and cooperative. Not all reports result in investigations. For example, you may have insufficient information about the alleged perpetrator for an investigation to go forward. The child abuse reporting laws tend to be constructed broadly in order to provide maximum protection for children, so they may capture situations such as those in which you have only minimal information about the abuse or where an investigation already is under way. Keep in mind that as a mandated reporter, you are not responsible for investigating or proving the suspected abuse.

Even if you are not mandated to report child abuse in a particular situation, nonetheless there may be clinical or ethical issues that need to be addressed. For example, if a child you are treating describes inappropriate physical contact by a neighbor and mandated reporting in your state is limited to situations in which the alleged abuser is a parent or legal guardian, you nevertheless will want to take action. In this case, you might decide to alert the child's parents and encourage them to take legal or other protective actions. You may also be in a unique position to help your patient and your patient's family by continuing therapy with the child and providing resources such as information about support groups to the parents. Another example of a situation that requires action other than reporting to a child abuse hotline is when you believe your patient or another person is in imminent danger of serious harm. In such cases, you may be permitted or mandated to release confidential information pursuant to the American Psychological Association Ethics Code Standard 4.05(b) and relevant state laws, including those governing the "duty to protect."

Ethics Code Standard 4.05(b) describes several situations in which disclosure of confidential information is allowed without patient consent, including "where permitted by law for a valid purpose such as to . . . protect the client/patient, psychologist, or others from harm." Further, the Health Insurance Portability and Accountability Act (HIPAA) Privacy Rule specifically permits covered health care providers to disclose reports of child abuse or neglect to public health authorities or other appropriate government authorities. These also are reiterated in several American Academy of Pediatrics and American Medical Association (AMA) Code of Ethics publications.

States also may differ regarding the reporting of past abuse. Most state laws or other guidelines clearly limit reportable situations to those involving children currently under the age of 18. For example, Washington's statute specifically states, "The reporting requirement . . . does not apply to the discovery of abuse or neglect that occurred during childhood if it is discovered after the child has become an adult. However, if there is reasonable cause to believe other children are or may be at risk of abuse or neglect . . . the reporting requirement . . . does apply" (Revised Code of Washington Title

26, 2020). Some state laws are unclear and could be interpreted as requiring a report even in cases of abuse alleged to have occurred many years ago.

If you are unsure about whether to report past abuse of a patient who is now an adult, you might consider contacting your state child protective services agency. A potentially complex situation arises when the abuse occurred in another state or the abuser now lives in another state. In such cases, contact your state's child protective services agency for advice. Your state's child protective services agency may be able to receive a report and coordinate investigative efforts with the other jurisdiction involved. You are unlikely to be mandated to report across state lines or permitted to release confidential information to another state's child protective services agency without your patient's consent. If you do need to make a report, it may make sense to discuss the situation with your patient and/or a minor patient's parents, even if you are allowed to make the report anonymously. The advisability of doing so will depend on factors such as the age of your patient, the nature of the family members' involvement, and clinical considerations. Explaining your legal obligations and emphasizing the goal of child protection may help to maintain the family's trust and enable you to continue in a therapeutic role.

Child abuse can trigger many emotions in the physician and the ED staff. Sadness and pity for the child and anger toward the parent or perpetrator often are exhibited. Staff members too upset by a particular situation should be relieved of the responsibility of working on that case.

In speaking with the patient, the righteousness of his or her decision to discuss abuse should be stressed. The patient might experience conflict about revealing a secret, especially a long-standing one that might or might not involve a family member or loved one. The patient often has a relationship with the perpetrator and realizes that this admission might alter their relationship. In most jurisdictions, sexual abuse is considered a criminal offense. Treatment issues, particularly protection of the child, require close cooperation between social services, medical services, and police. In the United States, sexual abuse of a child is a crime and requires reporting to the police. In many states, a specific statute requires that child sexual abuse be reported like all other child abuse to child protective services.

Child victims of sexual abuse face secondary trauma in the crisis of discovery. Their attempts to reconcile their private experiences with the realities of the outer world are assaulted by the disbelief, blame, and rejection they experience from adults. Dr. Roland C. Summit coined the phrase *Child Sexual Abuse Accommodation Syndrome* (CSAAS) in a paper written to describe the most typical reactions of children to abuse and to sensitize the criminal system to the legitimate victim of child abuse. The syndrome is separated into five categories that are said to epitomize the behavior of sexually abused children. Each element of the syndrome describes behavior that a child exhibits while adapting to an abusive situation. This is composed of the following five categories: secrecy, helplessness, entrapment and accommodation, delayed unconvincing disclosure, and retraction.

The first element, secrecy, indicates that the child will keep the abuse a secret and thereby allow it to continue. The authoritarian relationship between the abuser and the child also results in helplessness, the second element of CSAAS, which is exhibited by the child's continued tolerance of the abuse. As a result, the child must learn to accept the situation and thus accommodate the abuse in order to survive. Accommodation also may be exhibited through substance abuse, domestic martyrdom, distortion of reality, hysteria, sociopathy, and uncontrolled rage. In many sexual abuse cases involving children, disclosure is accomplished under suspicious circumstances. For example, in some cases, disclosure may be exposed by family conflict. If a family conflict induces disclosure, adults may discount the allegation as mere retaliation or rebelliousness. An adult may not believe that the abuse occurred over a period of many years. The golden rule in most child sexual abuse cases is that "whatever a child says about sexual abuse, s/he is likely to reverse it." This reaction often is a direct result of the pressure that the child must endure on disclosure. Disclosure forces the child to face both the disruption of the family unit and a legal system that often lacks sensitivity.

CASE RESOLUTION

Although the patient is an adult, you have concerns for her safety and well-being. Key is to ascertain if she still is subject to abuse by her father in her present living situation. After clarifying how the state laws apply, you explain to the patient your duty to ensure that she and others are not the targets of further abuse by her father. Despite your encouragement, the patient remains adamant that you not share the details of the sexual abuse. Because of her stated threats of self-harm, you initiate a mandatory psychiatric hold. It is your hope that she will pursue further counseling, if not legal action where appropriate, once afforded the opportunity by this admission.

KEY POINTS TO REMEMBER

- Statutes mandating physicians to report suspected cases of abuse can pose difficult dilemmas.
- These issues and situations often involve complicated legal, ethical, and interpersonal issues.
- It is important to be aware of the resources available to you within your institute, state, or national chapter of your professional organization.
- As hard as it is, sometimes situations or issues might not resolve the way you hope and intend. Give yourself some grace.

Suggested Reading

American Medical Association. Code of medical ethics. https://www.ama-assn. org/delivering-care/ethics/code-medical-ethics-overview. Accessed September 16, 2019.

American Psychological Association. APA code of ethics 2017, ethical principles of psychologists and code of conduct. https://www.apa.org/ethics/code/index. Accessed September 16, 2019.

Revised Code of Washington Title 26, Chapter 26.44, Section 26.44.030, https://app. leg.wa.gov/RCW/default.aspx?cite=26.44.030. Accessed February 1, 2020.

Section on Bioethics, American Academy of Pediatrics. Diekema DS, Leuthner SR, Vizcarrondo FE, eds. *American Academy of Pediatrics bioethics resident curriculum: case-based teaching guides*. Revised 2017.

Summit, C. Abuse of the child sexual abuse accommodation syndrome. *J Child Sex.* 1993 May 14; 1(4):153–164. doi:10.1300/j070v01n04_13.

11 The Drunken Drug Lord

Jeremy R. Simon

After stopping a car they saw driving erratically, police bring the uninjured driver, a 28-year-old male, into the emergency department (ED). They say that the patient has no medical complaints and did not want to come to the hospital, but they brought him regardless. They have no medical concerns either. However, they tell you that as they were approaching the car after they pulled it over, they believed they saw the patient place several items in his mouth and swallow them. Furthermore, the patient refused to take a breathalyzer test. The police request that you draw a blood alcohol level on the patient to see if he was driving under the influence. They also ask that you irrigate the patient's bowels so that they can recover the items he swallowed, which they think may be packets of drugs.

What do you do now?

LAW ENFORCEMENT IN EMERGENCY MEDICINE

Law enforcement agents most frequently arrive in the ED accompanying emotionally disturbed patients or prisoners with a medical complaint. In these cases, their role is merely that of an escort, passively observing the care of the patient (and assisting as needed) until we are able to release them back to other tasks. These cases create no dilemma for the emergency physician (EP) as there is no conflict between our ethical duty to act in the best interests of the patient and the police's law enforcement and public-order-maintaining responsibilities.

Occasionally, however, the police want us not only to treat their prisoner (or suspect), but also to assist in gathering evidence that might make a criminal case against our patient. Our case presents two of the most common requests police may make of the EP—performing tests on a patient and obtaining items such as contraband or bullets from the patient's body. These requests may create at least an apparent conflict with our duty to our patient and can be very stressful, especially if the police demand rather than request our assistance.

ETHICAL CONSIDERATIONS

As mentioned, our primary duty is always to act in our patient's best interests. Without this commitment, patients, especially from vulnerable populations, would not trust physicians and might avoid health care entirely. Such avoidance could ultimately create a large burden on society, so our commitment to patients' interests serves not only them but also society at large. There are exceptions, such as public health emergencies and certain violent crimes, where the patient's interests and society's differ so drastically that the law requires us, and medical ethics permits us, to place society's interests above the patient's. However, for such an exception to obtain, the benefit to society must be quite large. By and large, the patient's interests must guide our actions. Similarly, our obligation to maintain a patient's confidences is not absolute, but is a principle of medical ethics dating back to the Hippocratic oath.

LEGAL CONSIDERATIONS

The law also provides relevant guidance. Almost all states have legislation stating that anyone who drives in the state has implicitly consented to alcohol and drug testing, including blood, if the police deem it appropriate. The driver generally may refuse; however, often there are various penalties for this, such as loss of driver's license, fines, or even criminal charges.

Much of the relevant law, however, is case law and not legislation. The most relevant of these are six US Supreme Court cases: *Rochin v. California, Breithaupt v. Abram, Schmerber v. California, Missouri v. McNeely, Birchfield v. North Dakota,* and *Winston v. Lee.* In *Rochin,* police brought a patient to the ED whom they believed had swallowed narcotic capsules to hide. They asked that the capsules be retrieved. The physician placed an orogastric tube and administered an emetic, after which the patient regurgitated the capsules. The Supreme Court ruled that involuntarily "pumping" someone's stomach "shocks the conscience" and was a violation of due process.

By contrast, in *Breithaupt,* the court held that blood draws done on an unconscious patient to show that the suspect was driving while intoxicated are not problematic the same way "stomach pumping" is. *Schmerber* went even further and said that even blood drawn over a suspect's objections is admissible and does not need a search warrant because a blood draw is minimally invasive and the evidence (blood alcohol) will disappear. More recently, in *Missouri v. McNeely,* the Supreme Court clarified that whether or not concern for the metabolism of the alcohol counts as an emergency, obviating the need for a warrant, depends on the specific facts of the case, such as how long it has been since the driver was stopped. Finally (as of the time of this writing), in *Birchfield v. North Dakota,* the Supreme Court has said that although driving may be taken as implied consent for alcohol testing, it is not reasonable to say that a driver, by exercising his right to drive, has legally obligated himself, under threat of criminal penalties, to allow a blood alcohol test even if the police do not have a warrant.

Winston v. Lee deals with a somewhat different circumstance. In this case, Rudolph Lee attempted to rob a store and was shot by the shopkeeper. A bullet was lodged in his chest approximately 1 inch below the skin. The prosecutors in the case asked the court to force Lee to undergo surgery, under general anesthesia, so that the bullet could be recovered and used as evidence in the case against him. (Medically, there was no indication for removing the bullet.) When the case reached the Supreme Court, the court ruled that forcing a person to undergo surgery, unlike a simple blood draw, violates the right to be "secure in [one's] person" and that surgery cannot be compelled, even with a warrant.

One might ask why this extensive legal discussion is necessary. After all, what we are discussing here is the right thing to do, which is a matter of ethics, not what to do if we want to stay out of trouble with the law. In truth, the law often has a role in determining ethical behavior, for two reasons. First, as members of society, we (may) have an independent ethical obligation to obey the law, and this obligation will not be removed simply because it may conflict with another obligation, such as that to our patients. The proper resolution of such conflicts requires paying attention to all aspects of the situation and thus knowing the law. Second, as noted, the physician's duty to place patient interests, including confidentiality, above other competing interests derives at least in part from the value to society of our acting this way. Therefore, societal values and judgment, often expressed in law, are relevant to determining the strength of our obligations to our patients. Thus, for example, it is generally ethical and appropriate to comply with mandatory reporting laws even though they require us to violate patient confidentiality, usually for public health and safety reasons.

CASE RESOLUTION

Two general principles should govern all interactions with law enforcement. The American College of Emergency Physicians (ACEP) policy "Law Enforcement Information Gathering in the Emergency Department" states that acceding to a law enforcement request should never interfere with patient care. Unless legally obligated to do so, physicians should never release patient information without their consent, including their address or phone number. Furthermore, whenever one considers releasing information or evidence to the police, one should first contact the hospital's legal department. I am not a lawyer, and any legal conclusions one might derive from here must be confirmed.

Our case raises two particular issues, a blood draw and collection of contraband. Let us consider the blood draw first. Were our patient unconscious, we might be able to rely on implied consent, as discussed, although as of this writing, the US Supreme Court is considering if and when such implied consent laws apply to unconscious patients. (But see material that follows on whether one has a legal obligation to draw the test.) If the patient is conscious, implied consent no longer applies. If the conscious patient agrees to a test, then we may draw it. (We will not discuss here the impact that the patient's alcohol intake may have on his ability to consent to this.) Drawing the test for the police, even if there is no medical need, may even be seen as serving the patient's best interests, especially if we are drawing blood anyway, since if the physician does not draw the blood, the police will presumably have someone else do it, with a further needle-stick.

If the patient refuses, we are in a more difficult situation. Ethically, it would seem that the patient has the right to refuse, though it may result in their losing their license or other consequences, and that therefore we should not do the test. However, there is variation in what state laws require of physicians if the patient refuses to have blood drawn. Many states do not give any indication that healthcare professionals can be compelled to draw blood at the request of police. However, at least one state, Pennsylvania, requires physicians to draw blood samples for alcohol testing on all patients who are believed to be intoxicated and to have been involved in a motor vehicle crash, *even without* a police request. No allowance appears to be given for active patient refusal. Familiarity with local laws is essential in order to make an informed decision in this matter.

When it comes to retrieving drugs from our patient, the situation is clearer. There does not appear to be any state legislation obligating physicians to perform any sort of procedure to identify or obtain drugs or other contraband the patient may be hiding, even if the police have a warrant for allowing such a search. Some procedures, if done against the patient's will, may not be permitted even with a warrant. Only if such a procedure (e.g., a computed tomography scan, rectal examination, or bowel irrigation) is medically appropriate should it be done.

We must be careful in dealing with the drugs we *do* obtain from a patient, whether through therapeutic intervention or naturally, if the patient stays in the hospital long enough. Certainly, they must be disposed of in a legal manner, and this will often involve turning them over to law enforcement. However, this does not necessarily mean identifying the patient from whom they came if the police were not there at the time the drugs were retrieved (if, e.g., the patient was not under arrest at the time). Such information may well fall under physician-patient privilege, although one should certainly seek legal advice before asserting this privilege in the face of a court order or subpoena.

KEY POINTS TO REMEMBER

- Know all of the local laws and regulations, as well as hospital policies, regarding law enforcement requests.
- It is generally appropriate to comply with mandatory reporting laws.
- Collecting blood for police may be appropriate if the patient consents and in some states may be mandatory regardless.
- Physicians can generally not be compelled to do nonmedically appropriate searches for contraband in a patient.
- Disposing of contraband obtained from a patient must be done in a legal manner, and this may require involving the police. However, the identity of the patient the items were obtained from should generally remain confidential.
- When in doubt, contact hospital administration and its legal office early.

Suggested Reading

Baker EF, Moskop JC, Geiderman JM, et al. For the ACEP Ethics Committee. Law enforcement and emergency medicine: an ethical analysis. *Ann Emerg Med.* 2017;*68*:589–598.

Beauchamp RB. "Shed thou no blood": the forcible removal of blood samples from drunk driving suspects. *So Cal L Rev.* 1987;*60*;1115–1141.

Geiderman JM, Moskop JC, Derse AR. Privacy and confidentiality in emergency medicine: obligations and challenges. *Emerg Med Clin North Am.* 2006;*24*:633–656.

Law enforcement information gathering in the emergency department. *Ann Emerg Med.* 2017;*70*:942–943.

Malcolm KE, Malcolm JG, Wu DT, et al. Cops and docs: the challenges for ED physicians balancing the police, state laws, and EMTALA. *J Healthc Risk Manag.* 2017;*37*:29–35.

Moskop JC, Marco CA, Larkin GL, et al. From Hippocrates to HIPPA: privacy and confidentiality in emergency medicine—part I: conceptual, moral, and legal foundations. *Ann Emerg Med.* 2005;*45*:53–59.

Pilcher CA, Shroder E. Must an emergency physician comply with a body cavity search warrant? *ACEP Now.* 2016;*35*(10):13.

Rosen P, O'Connor M. The practice of medicine versus the practice of law. *J Emerg Med.* 1986;*4*:67–68.

Simon JR. Using physicians as agents of the state. In Jesus J, Grossman SA, Derse AR, Wolfe R, Adams JG, and Rosen P, eds., *Ethical problems in emergency medicine: a discussion-based review.* Malden, MA: Wiley-Blackwell; 2012:57–66.

12 No Country for Sick Men

Diane L. Gorgas and
Simiao Li-Sauerwine

Your charge nurse receives a call from a private dialysis clinic that a patient being treated there, Mr. R., was dismissed from the treatment center today because he was suspected of using a false ID. When confronted at the clinic, Mr. R. admitted to using his cousin's identification and insurance card because he is an undocumented citizen, but has renal failure and needs dialysis. The caller reports that Mr. R. received his complete treatment today, but that they suspect he may seek treatment at your hospital.

Shortly after entering a "patient expected" note in the electronic health record, a unit clerk comes to you and the charge nurse and reports she is concerned after overhearing one of the triage nurses saying he plans to call Immigration and Custom Enforcement when Mr. R. arrives.

What do you do now?

UNDOCUMENTED PERSONS

This case raises a series of ethical questions regarding the care of an undocumented person in the medical system, specifically in the emergency department (ED). First and foremost is the ethical dilemma about whether to report a suspected illegal immigrant to the Immigration and Naturalization Service (INS) or Immigration and Customs Enforcement (ICE), as the triage nurse has verbalized as his intention. Some medical staff believe that they have a duty to report, which is a fairly common belief among nonlawyers. However, both legally and ethically, there is no duty to report a crime, much less a suspected identity crime. In fact, once the patient is registered in the hospital system, including the act of providing his or her name and chief complaint, this personal information is protected by the Health Insurance Portability and Accountability Act (HIPAA). Reporting the patient would become a HIPAA violation unless (1) the information is used for health care treatment or billing, (2) Mr. R. gives his consent for his personal information to be given to government agencies, or (3) in very specific circumstances in which failure to report can constitute a public threat (communicable diseases, homicidal intent). No one from the ED may provide any information about the patient to immigration or law enforcement authorities, and the entire staff must protect his privacy from disclosure. A HIPAA breach can lead to substantial fines and penalties. The American College of Emergency Physicians' policy is in alignment with this stance, specifically opposing "federal and state initiatives which require physicians and health care facilities to refuse care to undocumented persons or to report suspected undocumented persons to immigration authorities" (American College of Emergency Physicians, 2018).

But, what is our obligation to treat? The ethical tenant of beneficence pertains to the physician's moral obligation to assess and treat any undocumented person. This is codified in the Emergency Medical Treatment and Active Labor Act (EMTALA) of 1986, which requires hospitals to provide a medically appropriate screening examination and any medically necessary stabilizing treatment for any patient who presents at the hospital's emergency department. The duty to screen and emergently treat the patient must occur independent of the provider's personal beliefs about the patient. Physicians cannot narrow categories of patients who deserve their care based on gender, race, ethnicity, sexual orientation, disease burden, or their socioeconomic or immigration status. Mr. R. must be assessed for medical stability, but assuming he is medically stable and completed his dialysis treatment prior to arrival, what is the provider's duty to ensure further treatment?

The standard of care for end-stage renal disease (ESRD) in the United States is three times weekly hemodialysis (HD) as a bridge to organ transplantation. Meeting this standard of care for undocumented patients has many practical and legal obstacles. By definition, undocumented persons are not eligible for government-provided health care coverage, including the Affordable Care Act (ACA). The Social Security Amendment of 1972 ensures access to kidney dialysis, but it is not available to undocumented persons. The cost of chronic HD for ESRD or renal transplantation is beyond the bounds of the vast majority of uninsured.

State-to-state variation about how to handle the care of chronically ill undocumented persons is enormous. Whereas some states will fund "maintenance dialysis" for undocumented persons, others will not, as was illustrated in the 2009 closing of Grady Memorial outpatient HD unit in Atlanta, Georgia, and the subsequent crisis resulting in abandonment of all its undocumented immigrant patients.

This disparity in access to care has led to divergent dialysis treatment strategies for undocumented ESRD patients, including (1) withholding routine treatment until symptoms develop. This reserves HD for "emergent" reasons, necessitating the ED as a point of care for these patients; (2) decreasing frequency of routine HD to weekly, or even longer, also termed *compassionate dialysis*; (3) providing the standard of care for treatment, but burdening beneficent health care organizations with the cost of providing that care; (4) recommendation for moving HD-dependent undocumented patients to states with more liberal funding for routine HD (California, Washington, New York); or (5) forced medical repatriation (deporting immigrants to their country of origin), where resources are severely lacking to provide chronic care. Further curtailing the options available is legal opinion (Connecticut State Court, Quiceno, 728 A.2 d. at 553 1999), which reads "fatal consequences of the discontinuance of ongoing [dialysis] care does not transform into emergency medical care." It is important to note that these proposed solutions either burden the patient with nonideal care, or no care, or increase financial stress on a medical system.

CASE RESOLUTION

Employing a health care organization's ethics service or an academic medical center's social medicine program can help define the duty of the institution to serve and provide some resources for logistics to accomplish the goals. Health care organizations should provide opportunities for all health care workers to discuss these challenges in a nonpunitive environment. Providing care for undocumented citizens creates an added ethical challenge to an already pressure-filled clinical setting, but is a dilemma that demands consideration in an increasingly complex health care landscape.

In our case, the ED physician, in conjunction with the unit supervisor, spoke to the unit clerk and emphasized that contacting authorities would represent a HIPAA violation, likely ending in disciplinary consequences for the employee. The unit clerk was referred to the hospital's Stress and Resiliency Employee program to discuss her dissatisfaction with the case in a nonpunitive and confidential environment. The patient's need for ongoing treatment was referred to the Compassionate Care Committee of the hospital, who set up regularly scheduled HD through the ED on a biweekly basis.

KEY POINTS TO REMEMBER

- There is not a duty to report undocumented citizens, and doing so may violate HIPAA regulations.
- EMTALA has been used as justification to provide care to undocumented citizens presenting to the ED seeking care options for chronic diseases.
- Alternative treatment regimens for undocumented citizens, such as delay of care or relocation of the patient, frequently do not provide ethically acceptable outcomes.
- Seek other institutional resources when confronted with the challenges of caring for undocumented citizens.

Suggested Reading

American College of Emergency Physicians. Policy statement, delivery of care to undocumented persons. Revised June 2018. https://www.acep.org/patient-care/policy-statements/delivery-of-care-to-undocumented-persons/. Accessed September 16, 2019.

Berlinger N. Is it ethical to bend the rules for undocumented and other immigrant patients? *AMA J Ethics*. 2019 Jan 1;*21*(1):E100–E105. doi:10.1001/amajethics.2019.100.

Quiceno v. Dept. of Social Services, 728 A.2d 553 (Conn. Super. Ct. 1999). https://www.courtlistener.com/opinion/3358750/quiceno-v-dept-of-social-services/

Rodriguez RA. Dialysis for undocumented immigrants in the United States. *Adv Chronic Kidney Dis*. 2015 Jan;*22*(1):60–65. doi: 10.1053/j.ackd.2014.07.003

Sacknov, K. Hospital falters as refuge for illegal immigrants. *New York Times*. November 20, 2019. https://www.nytimes.com/2009/11/21/health/policy/21grady.html. Accessed September 6, 2019.

Sconyers J, Tate T. How should clinicians treat patients who might be undocumented? *AMA J Ethics*. 2016 Mar 1;*18*(3):229–236. doi:10.1001/journalofethics.2016.18.3.ecas4-1603

13 The Reluctant Consultant

Sara R. Zaidi and Jeremy R. Simon

You are working at a rural, eight-bed emergency department (ED). The hospital provides some specialty surgery, including concerning ear, nose, and throat (ENT). At 2:00 a.m., a 27-year-old man presents with increasing throat pain over the past 24 hours. He reports chills and dysphagia, especially on the right. He has a temperature of 101.8°F, heart rate 115 beats per minute, blood pressure 128/87 mm Hg, and pulse oximetry of 97%. You note he has discomfort with swallowing, but is not drooling, and does not have true "hot potato" speech. You note swelling in the right peritonsillar area, and the uvula is slightly deviated. You suspect a peritonsillar abscess. Computed tomography (CT) of the neck soft tissues confirms edema without a drainable abscess. You initiate intravenous antibiotics and steroids.

You contact the ENT person on call and explain that the patient should be observed in case he deteriorates. The ENT refuses, saying that since there is no abscess he does not need admission to a surgical service. You do not think the patient should be admitted to the hospitalist because *if* he deteriorates, he will need an ENT.

What do you do now?

REFUSAL OF CARE (BY PROVIDERS TOWARD PATIENTS)

Emergency Medical Treatment and Active Labor Act and Legal Obligations

In order to discuss refusal of care in the ED, we must first discuss to whom we are obligated to provide care and in what situations. Congress passed the Emergency Medical Treatment and Active Labor Act (EMTALA) in 1986 in order to ensure that all patients with a medical emergency would be treated at any hospital to which they present or transferred to one that can. Specifically, anyone who presents to a hospital is entitled to a medical screening by a qualified medical provider to determine whether an emergency medical condition or active labor is present. An emergency medical condition is defined as any acute illness that left untreated would result in serious damage to the health of the patient or unborn child. If such a condition is present, medical stabilization must be provided regardless of the patient's ability to pay. Such stabilization includes any evaluation and treatment necessary to ensure that the patient's condition will not worsen when discharged. This may require admission to the hospital. If the hospital is unable to provide the services a patient needs, the hospital must make the patient stable for transport and arrange transfer to another hospital that can provide those services. A hospital with the available resources to treat a patient cannot refuse a transfer from another hospital that lacks those resources.

Prior to EMTALA, hospitals could refuse patients based on ability to pay, resulting in "dumping" of patients and their unreimbursed care onto other, often public, hospitals. With the advent of EMTALA, hospitals' participation in and reimbursement by Medicare became contingent on their being compliant with EMTALA's rules. Hospitals that violate EMTALA risk getting dropped from Medicare. Additionally, violations carry a steep monetary penalty; each infraction results in a fine for both the physician at fault and the hospital itself.

Furthermore, EMTALA applies not only to the emergency physicians (EPs) who do the initial treatment of patients, but also to any consultants who are needed to help stabilize and admit patients when needed. EMTALA requires hospitals to maintain a list of physicians who are on call to provide specialized services for any patient with an emergency medical condition who requires them for stabilization. (The hospital only has to provide on-call coverage for services they ordinarily provide.) While on call, a consultant cannot refuse to care for such patients even if they have no preexisting relationship with them because they are on call for the entire hospital. The consultant must also respond within a reasonable time. The on-call physician can send a representative (such as a resident physician or nurse practitioner) to evaluate the patient, but if the EP specifically requests that the on-call physician be present, the consultant has an obligation to come to evaluate the patient personally. If a hospital needs to transfer a patient because it does not have the resources to fully stabilize a patient, then an on-call consultant at a potential receiving hospital likewise must accept the patient, assuming the receiving hospital has the necessary resources to care for the patient.

One difference between an on-call doctor at the facility currently caring for the patient and one at a potential receiving hospital is that if the patient is currently in the consultant's hospital, the consultant must evaluate the patient if the EP insists, even if the consultant believes that he or she is not the appropriate specialist for the problem at hand. Since the EP remains responsible for the overall care of the patient until admitted, the EP is responsible for identifying the appropriate consultants. However, if the EP is attempting to transfer a patient to another hospital, the consultant would become responsible for the patient once the patient arrives and thus would be within his or her rights to refuse to accept a patient for whom the consultant did not feel equipped to care, even if the hospital as a whole could. The consultant should, however, direct the EP to the proper consultant at that hospital.

Under EMTALA, the hospital, EPs, and relevant consultants have an obligation to provide treatment only to the point that the emergency condition has been stabilized. There is no requirement for consultants to continue to provide outpatient care after the patient is stable and discharged.

A final point to note about EMTALA is that a failure to report to the government an EMTALA violation by someone else is, itself, an EMTALA violation, even if everything you did for the patient was both medically and legally appropriate.

Ethical Obligations

Regardless of its legal status, refusal by an on-call physician to come to evaluate a patient due to financial considerations, personal convenience, or discriminatory reasons violates an ethical obligation. By joining the on-call list, whether voluntarily or not, the physician has announced his or her willingness to provide care to anyone in need. This creates a double obligation for the on-call consultant. First, the consultant has directly obligated him- or herself to see the patients by saying that he or she would. Second, the consultant has indirectly obligated him- or herself by telling the other specialists who might have been on call, and perhaps would not have been reluctant to come in, that they do not need to be on call. By "sending away" these other potential providers, the on-call consultant has further obligated him- or herself to care for emergency patients.

The consultant cannot argue that these obligations are nullified because they were forced on him or her. There are many reasons why forced obligations still may be binding. In the case of physicians, one reason is particularly salient. Medical training, from medical school to residency, is a hugely complicated and expensive endeavor. No individual student or resident and no university or hospital can truly afford it or provide it on its own. They all require government subsidies. Thus, without government, that is, public, help, no one can become a physician. This support creates obligations. Whether those obligations are seen as being to the government or to the public, emergency stabilization of patients is the minimum that a society can expect in return for training physicians.

Additional Considerations

This is not to say that physicians, including consultants, can never refuse to treat a patient. Refusal of care if treatment violates physicians' religious or moral beliefs is a complex topic, and no concrete conclusions have yet been drawn. Federal legislation does allow doctors to refuse to give care that contradicts their moral or religious beliefs, though this has been challenged on multiple fronts. More straightforward is when physicians are asked to provide treatment that goes against good medical practice. In this case, they clearly have the right to refuse. Additionally, if a patient is violent or abusive, physicians have a right to ensure their own safety before treating such a patient.

Avoiding, Resolving, and Moving Beyond the Impasse

The first step is to be considerate and establish good working relationships. The ideal is cultivating a good rapport with consultants such that when you call for a consult, they wish to be helpful and do not question the validity of the patient's need. By avoiding calls during the night that can wait for a kinder hour, not overconsulting, and preferentially sending patients to clinic if possible, you can reserve consults for patients who have a truly emergent need. Good communication is also key to avoiding conflict. Make sure both you and the consultant have the relevant history and examination data. Be direct on the phone; explain why this is an emergency, what your question is, and why the consultant's services are needed.

Despite good relationships and communication, EPs sometimes encounter difficulties with consultants, who may refuse to come in to see or admit the patient or accept a transfer. In these situations, negotiation is the next step. Can the provider come in an hour or two to see the patient (assuming the EP is comfortable monitoring the patient somewhat longer)? Is there someone in the hospital under the consultant's supervision who can evaluate the patient directly and report back to him? If the consultant tells you that he or she does not want to come to see the patient because the consultant believes treatment should be provided by a physician of a different specialty, first try to understand this reasoning. Is there any test or study that can further delineate the appropriate specialty? Is the provider unable to offer the patient any treatment?

If negotiation fails, as the EP who is undertaking primary responsibility for the patient, if you still believe that the person you called is the appropriate specialist, then the specialist must come to see the patient to give formal and documented recommendations—even if the outcome of the evaluation is to state that there is no treatment that the specialist can offer. (A consultant at a potential receiving power has more autonomy, as the consultant must affirmatively accept a patient before the patient can be transferred.)

If you can come to no reasonable agreement, try an educational approach. Remind the provider of the on-call policy, and that the consultant risks violating EMTALA and incurring steep monetary fines, as well as exclusion of the hospital from Medicare/Medicaid plans if the consultant refuses to come in when directly requested to by the EP. If still you make no progress, then you must involve your hospital administrators to determine the next step. If the problematic consultant is at your own hospital, the next step may involve bringing in a second-call physician or transferring the patient to another hospital. There will be an EMTALA violation involved in transferring the patient because an available consultant would not come in. However, if, under the circumstances, the transfer is necessary for the patient's health, the violation will not be the EP's. Finally, remember that not reporting an EMTALA violation is itself a violation. If the consultant is at a potential receiving hospital, the decision may be made to contact administration at that hospital or transfer to another hospital, whichever would best serve the patient. Transfer to a different hospital also would involve an EMTALA violation, but not by your hospital.

CASE RESOLUTION

After you explain your concern about the need for an ENT if the patient deteriorates, the consultant still does not want to come in, saying the hospitalist can call him or her in that case, just as the nurse would if the patient were on his or her service. You agree to ask the hospitalist whether the hospitalist would be willing to accept the patient, but the hospitalist also is uncomfortable with a patient being admitted for a potential complication that would require a surgeon. When you call the ENT back to relay this, the consultant still sounds hesitant, so you remind the consultant of his or her obligations and your authority under the hospitals bylaws and their relationship to EMTALA, and she agrees to admit the patient.

KEY POINTS TO REMEMBER

· EMTALA obligates hospitals and the EPs on duty to provide a medical screening exam, and, if necessary, medical stabilization, to anyone who presents to an emergency department.
· Hospitals are required to have a roster of on-call specialists to assist in the stabilization of these patients as needed. These specialists are under the same EMTALA obligation to treat unstable patients as EPs.

- Although on-call specialists may be reluctant to come in to the hospital, especially during off hours, a collegial, considerate approach, with well-considered negotiation, will usually suffice to resolve the impasse.
- If the consultant absolutely will not come in, involve hospital administration to determine the next steps, which may include transferring the patient to another hospital. Make sure that the hospital reports the EMTALA violation, or you will also have committed one.

Suggested Reading

American College of Emergency Physicians (ACEP). EMTALA and on-call responsibility for emergency department patients. Policy statement. *Ann Emerg Med.* 2013;*62*:441–442.

Bitterman, RA. EMTALA and the ethical delivery of hospital emergency services. *Emerg Med Clin North Am.* 2006;*24*:557–577.

Hershey, N. EMTALA on-call coverage rule. *Hosp Law Newsl.* 2003;*21*:1–6.

Peth HA, Jr. The Emergency Medical Treatment and Active Labor Act (EMTALA): guidelines for compliance. *Emerg Med Clin North Am.* 2004;*22*:225–240.

14 Managing Bias and Belligerence

Shannon Markus and Carmen Wolfe

A 64-year-old white male with a history of hypertension (HTN), diabetes mellitus type 2, and hyperlipidemia presents to the emergency department (ED) via ambulance for chest pain. Emergency medical services (EMS) was called to his home a half hour ago when he began having substernal, pressure-like pain radiating to both shoulders. When you walk into the room, you note that the patient is diaphoretic and dyspneic. An electrocardiogram (ECG) shows inferior ST elevation consistent with ST-segment elevation myocardial infarction (STEMI). His heart rate is 105 beats per minute, but vital signs are otherwise normal. The patient is awake and alert and has a normal mental status.

As you introduce yourself, you notice tattoos on his arms, including a large swastika on his bicep. The patient ignores you—a female physician of color—and turns to the Caucasian nurse, asking for a new physician. He says that he wants "the best" doctor to care for him and will only accept treatment from a white male doctor. As you begin to address the patient, he raises his voice saying, "It's my *RIGHT* to choose my doctor! You can't force me to be treated by her!"

What do you do now?

THE RACIST OR BELLIGERENT PATIENT

A patient's racially motivated request for a provider reassignment raises difficult ethical and clinical questions. How do we balance a patient's autonomy and right to choose who cares for him or her with a provider's obligation to treat? How is this balance shifted in the special circumstance of a medical emergency?

Several ethical and practical factors must be considered when attempting to effectively balance patient preferences, employee rights, and the duty to treat. Determining the best course of action may vary depending on the patient's medical condition, his or her decision-making capacity, options for responding to the request, and specific reason for the request. Finally, the effect on the physician or staff member must also be considered as ensuring the safety of all team members is paramount.

EMERGENCY MEDICAL TREATMENT AND ACTIVE LABOR ACT

The first consideration in this patient's case is that of clinical acuity and potential instability. Patients presenting with an emergency medical condition are protected by the Emergency Medical Treatment and Active Labor Act (EMTALA), which mandates that Medicare-participating hospitals and other health care centers provide stabilizing treatments before arranging appropriate transfer, if warranted, for a variety of medical conditions, regardless of a person's citizenship, legal status, or ability to pay. In an emergency situation where the patient is unstable, the patient should be treated promptly and stabilized, regardless of expressed racial preferences. If an emergency medical condition can be ruled out quickly, then the patient may be discharged and choose to receive follow-up care with any provider according to his or her preferences. The gray area lies in situations where patients are stable enough to express their preferences, but their presentation represents an emergent medical condition requiring immediate treatment.

DECISION-MAKING CAPACITY

Assessing a patient's decision-making capacity represents a key step in determining how to proceed when confronted with these situations. Patients with unstable vital signs or altered mental status may not be able to make sound decisions, including the decision to decline care based on race, gender, or other characteristics of their provider. In these cases, emergent treatments should be provided until the patient is determined to have decision-making capacity, at which point the team may return to address the patient's requests. Decision-making capacity may vary with time or vary based on the specific decision to be made and may only be temporarily suspended in cases of delirium or other reversible disorders. Forceful provision of care to an unwilling patient who has capacity to decline, even if deemed to be beneficial, may be considered battery, a criminal offense and a basis for civil cases as well.

CULTURAL CONFLICT—EXPLORING THE RATIONALE BEHIND THE REQUEST

While this case vignette offers an example of obvious bigotry based on racist remarks insinuating the inferiority of one race and sex to another, there may be times when more appropriate requests regarding physician staffing may be made by patients. If not explicitly offered by the patient, the physician should seek to understand the reasoning behind a patient's request. Efforts should be made first to explore the patient's concerns without the immediate intention of changing the patient's mind. This constructive response to discrimination may identify specific reasons for the patient's request such as fears or misconceptions that can in turn be addressed without requiring a provider substitution. In some cases, the physician may be able to reassure a patient regarding his or her qualifications to expertly treat a patient, such as a patient who requests an allopathic physician instead of an osteopathic physician. In other cases, the physician may discover that a request for a specific gender physician stems from well-established religious concerns, such as the request of a Muslim woman not to be examined by a male physician. Exploring these reasons with open-ended questions gives the patient an opportunity to express his or her concerns and may help to explain a seemingly sexist, racist, or otherwise exclusionary request.

NEGOTIATION OR ACCOMMODATION

A provider may choose to approach the situation by using negotiation and persuasion, with the goal of coming to a mutually acceptable agreement with the patient that allows the physician to provide appropriate medical care. One strategy to consider employing is cultivating a therapeutic alliance by building rapport, exploring biases, and redirecting the conversation to that of the patient's current illness and medical care. While medical education does not typically include significant instruction on initiating appropriate dialogue between physicians and patients about patient-held biases, the ability to lead such a conversation is an invaluable skill. By focusing on the medical issues at hand and drawing attention to the need for emergent intervention, providers may be able to refocus a patient's attention to their health emergency and look past their biases in order to receive prompt care.

If these strategies are unsuccessful and the patient requires acute medical care, the provider can discuss with their physician colleagues the option to accommodate the patient's request to switch providers. Occasionally, accommodation is possible, especially in the case of multiple provider coverage, as is often seen in larger emergency departments. Providers may decide among themselves if a physician reassignment is reasonable, is logistically sound, and will not negatively affect patient care for the individual or for other patients in the ED. While accommodating such a request may feel like acquiescing and therefore condoning a patient's racist behavior, there are some potential benefits of accommodation. Racially concordant patient-doctor relationships have been shown in several studies to be more effective, with higher patient satisfaction and better health outcomes than racially discordant relationships. This decision to accommodate lies with the physicians on service and may not be possible in times of single coverage. In the case that accommodation is not an option, the physician may wish to explore the possibility of transferring the patient to a different facility if further evaluation or treatment is necessary for an emergent medical condition.

Regardless of the outcome to negotiate or accommodate, providers should strictly limit unacceptable conduct. Specific guidelines and expectations should be set, and patients should be informed that racist, discriminatory, and hateful speech is unacceptable. In the case of a stable patient without a life-threatening emergency who continues to employ discriminatory speech or actions with a refusal to yield, it is reasonable to dismiss the patient from the health care setting.

THE BELLIGERENT PATIENT AND STAFF SAFETY

During the course of negotiating with patients in these difficult situations, physicians may find themselves faced with a patient whose behavior escalates from belligerent remarks into physical violence. Multiple studies have demonstrated the alarmingly high rates of workplace violence toward ED employees, and in cases of escalating patient violence, it is paramount to maintain staff safety. Prevention of these situations may be accomplished by noting the warning signs of escalating behavior. Verbal deescalation techniques can be employed by staff members to diffuse a potentially escalating situation. Pharmacologic interventions may be offered voluntarily to a patient whose behavior spirals out of control. Finally, involuntary pharmacologic intervention or, as a last resort, physical restraint may be required to maintain staff safety. By proactively identifying escalating behavior, physicians can hope to avoid these more extreme measures.

IMPACT ON PHYSICIANS

According to Title VII of the 1964 Civil Rights Act, employees of health care institutions have the right to a workplace protecting them from discrimination based on race, color, or national origin. Despite this protection, physicians often find themselves subject to discrimination, wrestling between their desire to provide the standard of care to a patient regardless of their racist beliefs and the moral injury that being the subject of this discrimination may cause. Mistreatment extends to trainees as well, with studies revealing this as a widespread phenomenon, identifying discrimination based on gender and race as most prevalent. In addition to potential physical injury, many minority providers faced with such requests targeted at their gender, race, or ethnicity endure moral injury as well. Patients' refusal of care from these physicians can be humiliating and demoralizing and eventually can lead to burnout. Care must be taken to adequately address patient requests for a different provider that are motivated by bigotry in a way that protects and uplifts the physician while not compromising patient safety.

CASE RESOLUTION

You recognize that your patient is facing a life-threatening condition and take a moment to consider how to strike a careful balance between the patient's autonomy and your duty to treat him. Despite the discriminatory comments made by the patient, you calmly introduce yourself as the physician on duty, sit down at the bedside, and verbalize your genuine commitment to caring for him. The patient grumbles in dissatisfaction and repeats his request for another provider. You emphasize that you are the only physician available in the ED and are the most qualified person to take care of him. You begin to focus on his medical concerns and steer the conversation toward the acuity of his condition, with the need for immediate intervention for his heart attack. Explaining the need to act quickly to reduce his long-term morbidity, you offer him options of continuing under your care or requesting transfer to a different facility, which might be associated with a significant delay in his care. You remain calm, demonstrate your genuine concern for the patient, and wait patiently for him to make a choice given that his capacity to make medical decisions is intact. As he continues to deliberate, you encourage him to call a family member to help him talk through this decision, and his wife uses her concern for his health to successfully convince him to accept the care that you are offering to provide. You enlist the help of your charge nurse to engage in a discussion on acceptable behaviors to proceed with care in a mutually respectful environment so that the patient's discriminatory remarks do not affect any other staff members and to prevent any escalation of unacceptable behaviors.

- Patients who are unstable or who lack decision-making capacity should be stabilized before considering any discriminatory request for provider reassignment.
- Exploration of the patient's rationale behind his or her request through thoughtful dialogue may resolve biases or reveal reasonable culturally appropriate explanations.
- If negotiation fails to identify a middle ground that allows for optimal patient care, consideration may be made to accommodate a request depending on the resources available within the department or to offer transfer.
- Belligerent behavior should be managed with verbal deescalation and show of force, followed by pharmacologic therapies if the safety of the patient or providers is threatened.

Suggested Reading

Chen P. When the patient is racist. *The New York Times*. July 25, 2013. https://well. blogs.nytimes.com/2013/07/25/when-the-patient-is-racist/. Accessed July 1, 2019.

Novick D. Racist patients often leave doctors at a loss. *The Washington Post*. October 19, 2017. https://www.washingtonpost.com/opinions/racist-patients-often-leave-doctors-at-a-loss/2017/10/19/9e9a2c46-9d55-11e7-9c8d-cf053ff30921_story.html. Accessed July 1, 2019.

Paul-Emile K. Patients' racial preferences and the medical culture of accommodation. *UCLA Law Rev*. 2012;*60*:462–504.

Paul-Emile K, Smith AK, Lo B, Fernández, A. Dealing with racist patients. *N Engl J Med*. 2016;*374*(8):708–711.

Whitgob EE, Blankenburg RL, Bogetz AL. The discriminatory patient and family: strategies to address discrimination towards trainees. *Acad Med*. 2016;*91*(11):S64–S69.

Ziaei M, Massoudifar A, Rajabpour-Sanati A, Pourbagher-Shahri AM, Abdolrazaghnejad A. Management of violence and aggression in emergency environment; a narrative review of 200 related articles. *Adv J Emerg Med*. 2018;*3*(1):e7.

15 Very Important Patients

Kelsey Nestor and Carmen Wolfe

As the emergency department (ED) physician on the Monday after Thanksgiving, you are busy, with all of your rooms occupied and an overflowing waiting room. You receive a call from the hospital chief executive officer (CEO) that his friend, a prominent hospital donor, will be arriving soon by private vehicle for evaluation after stepping on a nail. The CEO has arranged to open up one of your rooms for this VIP and asks you to attend to him immediately given his past donations. Prior to the VIP's arrival, your waiting room triage nurse expresses her concerns about a patient with sickle cell disease who is presenting with acute chest pain. The patient is well known to you and has frequent ED visits, but his oxygen saturations are 93% on room air, which isn't typical for him. Your only evaluation and treatment space is the room earmarked for the VIP, and it's unlikely that another space will open soon. You know that the CEO will be upset if his VIP donor has to wait while his room is given to a "frequent flier."

What do you do now?

INTERPERSONAL AND INSTITUTIONAL CONFLICT

In the ED, we pride ourselves on taking care of anyone at any time. Our moral charge applies not only to uninsured or disadvantaged patients, but also to those on the other side of this spectrum. These "VIPs" represent a special population, named as such for the common abbreviation for very important people, though in the hospital setting, they probably are more accurately described as very intimidating patients. Although popular culture would traditionally identify VIPs as universally known celebrities such as famous singers, actors, government officials, athletes, notorious criminals, or authors, another category of VIPs also merits specific discussion. These special individuals are not as well known, but their lack of universal name recognition is eclipsed by their spheres of influence. While these individuals would simply be regular patients at another facility, their roles place them in VIP status at a specific institution. Hospital administrators, department staff members, fellow physicians, and, as in this case, hospital donors, all merit VIP status given the preferential considerations made on their behalf in the ED.

Despite the often-stated goal to treat all patients equally, an honest assessment of your own personal practice patterns likely includes providing preferential treatment to VIPs that deviates from routine care in some way. While this preferential treatment may refer specifically to the medical care they receive, it may also simply reflect a deviation in triage, reserving special rooms, or moving someone up in the queue to be seen out of usual order. A Connecticut College of Emergency Physicians survey of medical directors from 33 hospitals in Connecticut asked this very question, and all but one director endorsed providing different treatment for VIP patients in the ED. Beyond deviations in medical care or triage order, some hospitals now even offer deluxe suites and VIP floors to patients who are able and willing to pay for these specialized services. Evaluation of 15 well-known hospitals in the United States revealed that 10 of these offered some variation of these optional luxury treatment options.

Special Attention

There's no denying that VIPs often receive, at the very least, different medical care than the general population. This subject hits close to home for many physicians who may have enjoyed the benefits of these unwritten policies. Perhaps the physician or a family member has found himself or herself placed in a private room rather than a hallway stretcher. An advanced imaging test may be facilitated in the ED rather than deferred to the outpatient setting. A personal cell phone number for a specialist is given out for any follow-up concerns or questions. These small conveniences add up to an improved experience for VIPs, all predicated on favors done for colleagues. But is this the right thing to do? Are VIPs receiving better care overall?

A paramount concern when caring for a VIP is maintaining patient privacy. With celebrities, athletes, and political figures comes an onslaught of media attention as well as eager medical staff who want to be involved. Efforts to maintain their right to privacy must be much more aggressive, as they can be easily recognized in waiting rooms, in hallways, and on whiteboard displays. Efforts to maintain privacy often require additional services, such as increased security or use of portable imaging, though these additional resources of time, effort, and cost are ethically justified to ensure that VIPs have the same level of privacy as the general population. It is important for hospital administration to be transparent to both staff and other patients regarding the rationale for this preferential treatment, explaining that the resources are being directed toward preserving privacy so as to not lose the trust of other patients and staff members. In these extreme cases, rooming a VIP from the waiting room more expeditiously may be warranted to preserve their privacy, justifying a deviation from traditional triage order.

Although privacy concerns may not be paramount for those whose names or faces are not immediately recognizable, local VIPs such as the hospital donor in this vignette often find themselves with more staff involved in their care than typical patients. This element of "too many cooks in the kitchen" arises as staff may consider caring for a VIP to be an opportunity for advancement or recognition, giving them access to restricted information. Often, department chairs and upper level administrators may try to insert themselves in the patient's care teams, requesting frequent updates, asking for specific tests or procedures to be ordered, or coming in to take care of the patient themselves. Shielding the patient from this well-intentioned attention may be necessary to preserve their privacy. Restricting information may feel difficult when these requests for updates come from physicians or administrators in positions of authority. If unnecessary to facilitate patient care, and if unrequested by the patient, these sidebar updates should never be provided. Privacy is a basic right of the patient and every effort should be made to safeguard this right.

Though one might presume that expediting care of a VIP is unfair to other patients, some argue that providing special treatment to a VIP may motivate them to donate money or resources to the department, which ultimately may benefit all patients. In contrast, others suggest that providing VIPs with more typical experiences by having them wait in the waiting room or be placed in a hallway bed may be a stimulus for change and progress at the administrative level. Perhaps a VIP who waits for a workup for many hours in a hallway bed would be motivated to advocate for funding more examination rooms in an ED. Paramount to both of these arguments, however, is the importance of providing quality care in a timely manner to the VIP. Although the VIP often has power and influence that far exceed that of the hospital staff, it is important to remain mindful that this actually makes them a very vulnerable population. Making health care decisions based on their influence violates their rights to equal care, even if the primary motivation is theoretically to provide better care for all.

Perils of Special Treatment

Although never formally studied and despite popular belief, many speculate that VIPs actually receive inferior care compared to typical patients. Physicians and staff may alter their normal operating procedures in order to avoid inconveniencing a VIP or may pursue exceedingly aggressive therapies or workups in order to avoid missing pathology. The pressure and sheer awe of taking care of a VIP can paralyze even the best clinicians, creating a particularly dangerous scenario in the ED, where we frequently need to treat life-threatening illnesses in a systematic and expedited manner. For gray areas in medical decision-making, physicians may find themselves in a place of indecision and erroneously rely on the VIP to make this decision rather than using their best judgment. This phenomenon is most often seen when the VIP is a physician, as the treating physician may wish to please the patient by giving the patient more independence than the general population. This deviation from normal behavior may stem from the physician's desire to please the patient or to defer blame if the wrong choice is determined to have been made in retrospect. It is our responsibility as physicians to take responsibility for the care of our patients, and efforts must be made to maintain the roles of patient and physician, removing the burden of decision from the patient and optimizing their outcome.

Another factor contributing to inferior care for VIPs lies in the hesitancy of physicians to perform a complete history and physical examination. Physicians may find themselves reluctant to fully disrobe a patient or deferring invasive portions of the examination, such as pelvic or rectal exams. In an effort to avoid embarrassing or offending VIPs, physicians may omit questions about psychiatric or substance abuse history. These difficult questions may provide key elements necessary for accurate diagnosis and treatment, and by avoiding seemingly invasive yet appropriate questions, there is a large potential to miss out on critical diagnoses. By redoubling efforts to equalize treatment of all patients and continuing a uniform approach to each patient encounter, physicians can avoid this critical pitfall.

Finally, maintaining the usual care team structure for VIPs also will help to prevent deviations from standard care. VIPs often find themselves attracting the personal care of department chiefs or other physician leaders and are less likely to have residents or students involved in their care. Department leaders often become involved in the care of VIPs due to a personal request or a perceived expectation to be involved in high-profile cases, rather than because of the specific clinical expertise that they can provide. As leaders in their fields, they may be removed from the practicalities of day-to-day functionality of the hospital, which may hinder the clinical care of the patient. Furthermore, while VIPs or their surrogates may decline involvement of trainees in their care, it is recommended that trainees play an active role in the care of VIPs. This preservation of the standard team structure ensures the same quality of care that is provided for every other patient. Trainees also are well versed in the inner workings of the hospital, and their involvement may be advantageous to the patient's care by expediting certain processes. Because deviation from standard of care is a major factor leading to poorer outcomes in VIPs, every effort should be made to preserve a typical care team structure.

Having self-awareness of the increased likelihood of providing different medical care is crucial to providing these patients with equal medical care. Health care providers should continually question and reevaluate if they are providing the standard of care to this potentially vulnerable population. Becoming aware of our own internal biases and actively working to oppose these biases will ultimately make us better physicians.

CASE RESOLUTION

You place the frequent flier with sickle cell crisis and hypoxia in the only available room, as reprioritizing care for this VIP would violate your ethical duty to fairness. You confidently inform your hospital CEO that the donor will receive the best possible care, which centers on treating the VIP just like any other patient. You emphasize the need to maintain usual triage standards in order to avoid compromising the care of other critically ill patients. You meet with the donor to explain the delay and assure him that his privacy will be maintained during his ED visit. When asked about the wait, you assure him that triage and treatment according to standard protocol will ensure that he obtains the best possible health outcomes. He thanks you for your attention and commends you on the hard work you are doing to fairly treat all patients in the most efficient manner possible.

KEY POINTS TO REMEMBER

- Standard triage should be used to determine treatment order for VIPs unless this practice would violate their privacy or cause disruption in the department.
- Beware of the tendency to omit sensitive questions or physical examinations that might embarrass a VIP, as this may lead to lapses in care.
- Avoiding deviation from routine care is critical in achieving the best outcomes for VIPs.

Suggested Reading

Clarke SA. How hospitals coddle the rich. *NY Times*, October 26, 2015. https://www.nytimes.com/2015/10/26/opinion/hospitals-red-blanket-problem.html. Accessed June 1, 2019.

Groves JE, Dunderdale BA, Stern TA. Celebrities, VIPs and potentates primary care companion. *J Clin Psychiatry*. 2002;*4*(6):215–223.

Guzman JA, Sasidhar M, Stoller JK. Caring for VIPs: nine principles. *Clev Clin J Med*. 2011;*78*:90–94.

Schenkenberg T, Kochenour NK, Botkin JR. Ethical considerations in clinical care of the "VIP." *J Clin Ethics*. 2007;*18*(1):56–63.

Smally AJ, Carroll B, Carius M, Tilden F, Werdmann M. Treatment of VIPs. *Ann Emerg Med*. 2011;*58*(4):397–398.

Smith MS, Shesser RF. The emergency care of the VIP patient. *N Engl J Med*. 1988;*319*(21):1421–1423.

16 Frequent Flyer

Catherine A. Marco

A 32-year-old woman presents to the emergency department (ED) with symptoms of abdominal discomfort, nausea, and vomiting. She has had numerous ED visits for similar symptoms. She has had five abdominal computed tomographic (CT) scans in the past 2 months. She states, "The pain is a 12! It feels like my bowel obstruction. I need a CT scan. And dilaudid is the only thing that works for me."

What do you do now?

STEWARDSHIP OF HEALTH CARE RESOURCES

Stewardship of health care resources is an important bioethical tenet of the practice of medicine. Physicians should act as stewards of resources, and ensure that they are appropriately used to provide the best possible medical care for individual patients and for society as a whole.

Health care costs in the United States are among the highest in the world. The costs of health care are complex and multifactorial. Some of the driving forces include price of drugs, medical devices, hospital care, taxes, hospital administration, and insurance administration. Several studies have demonstrated that physicians are poor at estimating the costs of laboratory and radiographic tests.

The American College of Emergency Physicians (ACEP, 2019) has stated in ACEP's Code of Ethics for Emergency Physicians, "emergency physicians shall act as responsible stewards of the health care resources entrusted to them." The Code of Ethics expounds:

> Both society and individual emergency physicians confront questions of justice in deciding how to distribute the benefits of health care and the burdens of financing that care among the various members of the society. Emergency physicians routinely address these issues when they assign order of priority for treatment and choose appropriate diagnostic and treatment resources. In making these judgments, emergency physicians must attempt to reconcile the goals of equitable access to health care and just allocation of health care with the increasing scarcity of resources and the need for cost containment. (ACEP, 2017a: 11)

Similarly, the American Medical Association (AMA, 2019) has stated in the "Physician Stewardship of Health Care Resources,"

> Physicians' primary ethical obligation is to promote the well-being of individual patients. Physicians also have a long-recognized obligation to patients in general to promote public health and access to care. This obligation requires physicians to be prudent stewards of the shared societal resources with which they are entrusted. Managing health care resources responsibly for the benefit of all patients is

compatible with physicians' primary obligation to serve the interests of individual patients.

Stewardship of resources requires the appropriate use of diagnostic and therapeutic interventions that will be of benefit to the patient and the avoidance of unnecessary or costly interventions that will not improve outcome. Decisions about health care resources should be made based on beneficence and benefit to the patient and not on economic or social standing, ability to pay, worthiness, or other judgmental issues.

Specific interventions to reduce the cost of emergency care include considering and limiting costs of laboratory tests, high-cost imaging, medications, intravenous fluids and medications, hospital admissions, and postdischarge care.

In an effort to promote wise stewardship of medical resources, the Choosing Wisely campaign was launched in 2011 by the ABIM Foundation. Over 80 medical societies and consumer groups have participated, including ACEP, to promote communication between physicians and patients about appropriate tests and treatments and avoiding care when harm may outweigh benefits. ACEP's recommendations are listed in Table 16.1.

The question may arise, should the physician act only in the best interest of the individual patient or in the best interest of society? ACEP (2019) has stated in "Clinical Policy: Emergency Physician Stewardship of Finite Resources"

> The best medical interest of the patient should be foremost in any clinical decision making process. Criteria for appropriate use of finite resources should include (1)urgency of the patient's medical condition; (2) likelihood, magnitude, and duration of medical benefit to the patient; (3) burdens and costs of care to the patient; and (4) cost to society.

Rationing of health care resources may be necessary for scarce or expensive therapies. Although rationing is often necessary in developing countries, widespread availability of technology and therapies in the United States does not often lead to rationing. However, unfettered health care spending may limit resource availability in the future, and rationing may become necessary.

TABLE 16.1 **Choosing Wisely: American College of Emergency Physicians**

Eight Things Physicians and Patients Should Question

1. Avoid computed tomographic (CT) scans of the head in emergency department patients with minor head injury who are at low risk based on validated decision rules.

2. Avoid placing indwelling urinary catheters in the emergency department for either urine output monitoring in stable patients who can void or patient or staff convenience.

3. Don't delay engaging available palliative and hospice care services in the emergency department for patients likely to benefit.

4. Avoid wound cultures in emergency department patients with uncomplicated skin and soft tissue abscesses after successful incision and drainage and with adequate medical follow-up.

5. Avoid instituting intravenous (IV) fluids before doing a trial of oral rehydration therapy in uncomplicated emergency department cases of mild-to-moderate dehydration in children.

6. Avoid CT of the head in asymptomatic adult patients in the emergency department with syncope, insignificant trauma, and a normal neurological evaluation.

7. Avoid CT pulmonary angiography in emergency department patients with a low pretest probability of pulmonary embolism and either a negative Pulmonary Embolism Rule-Out Criteria (PERC) or a negative D-dimer.

8. Avoid lumbar spine imaging in the emergency department for adults with nontraumatic back pain unless the patient has severe or progressive neurologic deficits or is suspected of having a serious underlying condition (e.g., such as vertebral infection, cauda equina syndrome, or cancer with bony metastasis).

ETHICAL CONSIDERATIONS

Autonomy

Respect for patient autonomy refers to respect for an individual's right to make medical decisions about his or her own body. Providers should respect the right of patients to make medical decisions that reflect their own goals and values. Decisions should be based on clear and accurate information and should be free of coercion. However, respect for patient autonomy is not absolute and does not allow the patient to dictate unreasonable interventions.

Every attempt should be made to come to a mutually agreeable course of action to diagnose and treat the patient's condition. If agreement cannot be reached, the physician is not obligated to provide care that is contrary to his or her professional judgment or moral beliefs. ACEP (2017b) has stated in policy: *Physicians are not obligated to provide treatment that in their professional judgment, have no realistic likelihood of benefit to the patient.*

Beneficence

Beneficence, the obligation to act in the best interest of patients, applies to this decision. The provider has a duty to do good or to promote the patient's welfare. As in all shared decision-making, the physician should recommend the best diagnostic and treatment regimen and offer a discussion with the patient about risks, benefits, and how this fits with the patient's goals and values.

Nonmaleficence

Nonmaleficence, the obligation to not inflict harm intentionally, has application in this case. Nonmaleficence often references the phrase *primum non nocere* ("first, do no harm"). This principle mandates that the provider should avoid any action that would intentionally harm the patient. In this case, the risks of excessive unnecessary radiation and cost may outweigh the negligible diagnostic benefit of a repeat diagnostic CT scan.

Justice

Justice, the duty of fairness in processes and distribution of benefits, applies to this case. Justice includes three categories: distribution of scarce resources, respect for patient's rights, and respect for morally acceptable laws. Some diagnostic or therapeutic interventions may be expensive, labor intensive, or resource intensive. Such interventions should be carefully considered by physicians and patients to ensure their appropriate use in a specific case. Although stewardship of resources is important in a global sense, in general, the high cost of a specific treatment should not influence the care of an individual patient if proven to be efficacious.

CASE RESOLUTION

As in all cases of the physician-patient relationship, goals of therapy should be delineated, and appropriate diagnostic and therapeutic interventions to achieve that goal should be undertaken. In most cases, physician and patients agree with the same goal of improving patient comfort and health. However, at the same time, there may be discordance between patient and physician. Shared decision-making should be undertaken to elicit the patient's goals and values and then to educate and inform the patient about the physician's recommendations. The goal is to reach a mutually agreeable course of action based on the patient's goals and values. If unable to reach agreement, the physician should offer the tests and therapy that offer the best good to the patient. Tests that are expensive and potentially harmful should not be offered simply because the patient requests them.

KEY POINTS TO REMEMBER

- Physicians have a duty to use health care resources wisely.
- Physicians and patients should establish goals of therapy.
- Appropriate diagnostic and therapeutic interventions should be undertaken.
- Shared decision-making is an important component of medical decision-making.
- Emergency physicians should order tests and therapies that promote patient health and well-being.
- Unnecessary, expensive, or potentially harmful interventions should not be done, even at the patient's request.

Suggested Reading

American College of Emergency Physicians. Five things physicians and patients should question. 2015. Available at: http://www.choosingwisely.org/wp-content/uploads/2015/02/ACEP-Choosing-Wisely-List.pdf. Accessed March 2, 2019.

American College of Emergency Physicians. Code of Ethics form Emergency Physicians. 2017a. Available at: https://www.acep.org/globalassets/new-pdfs/policy-statements/code-of-ethics-for-emergency-physicians.pdf?_t_id=ejTCR_h2YnHxDpp7JayjEw==&_t_q=code%20of%20ethics&_t_tags=andquerymatch,language:en%7Clanguage:7D2DA0A9FC754533B091FA6886A51C0D,sitei

d:3f8e28e9-ff05-45b3-977a-68a85dcc834a%7Csiteid:84BFAF5C52A349A0BC61
A9FFB6983A66&_t_ip=&_t_hit.id=ACP_Website_Application_Models_Media_
DocumentMedia/_bea22949-bb55-4462-83d0-7a56dbb9c623&_t_hit.pos=0.
Accessed February 2, 2020.

American College of Emergency Physicians. Nonbeneficial ("futile") emergency
medical interventions. Revised 2017b. Available at: https://www.acep.org/patient-
care/policy-statements/nonbeneficial-futile-emergency-medical-interventions/.
Accessed February 28, 2019.

American College of Emergency Physicians. Emergency physician stewardship of
finite resources. 2019. Available at: https://www.acep.org/globalassets/new-pdfs/
policy-statements/emergency-physician-stewardship-of-finite-resources.pdf.
Accessed February 19, 2019.

American College of Emergency Physicians. Resource utilization in the emergency
department: the duty of stewardship. n.d. Available at: https://www.acep.org/
globalassets/new-pdfs/preps/resource-utilization-in-the-emergency-department---
the-duty-of-stewardship---prep.pdf. Accessed February 28, 2019.

American Medical Association Code of Medical Ethics. Code of medical
ethics: consent, communication & decision making. n.d. Available at: https://
www.ama-assn.org/delivering-care/ethics/code-medical-ethics-consent-
communication-decision-making. Accessed February 28, 2019.

American Medical Association Code of Medical Ethics. Physician stewardship of
health care resources. n.d. Available at: https://www.ama-assn.org/delivering-
care/ethics/physician-stewardship-health-care-resources. Accessed February
28, 2019.

Barry MJ, Edgman-Levitan S. Shared decision making—the pinnacle of patient-
centered care. *N Engl J Med*. 2012;*366*(9):780–781.

Cutler DM. Rising medical costs mean more rough times ahead. *JAMA*. 2017 Aug
8;*318*(6):508–509.

Hess EP, Grudzen CR, Thomson R, et al. Shared decision-making in the emergency
department: respecting patient autonomy when seconds count. *Acad Emerg
Med*. 2015;*22*:856–864.

Krauss CK, Marco CA: Shared decision-making in the emergency department: ethical
considerations. *Am J Emerg Med*. 2016 Aug;*34*(8):1668–1672.

Long T, Silvestri MT, Dashevsky M, Halim A, Fogerty RL. Exit survey of senior
residents: cost conscious but uninformed. *J Grad Med Educ*. 2016
May;*8*(2):248–251.

Lynn D, Knoedler MA, Hess EP, et al. Engaging patients in health care decisions in the
emergency department through shared-decision making: a systematic review.
Acad Emerg Med. 2012;*19*:959–967.

Maughan BC, Baren JM, Shea JA, et al. Choosing wisely in emergency medicine: a
national survey of emergency medicine academic chairs and division chiefs.
Acad Emerg Med. 2015 Dec;*22*(12):1506–1510.

Sarela AI. Stop sitting on the fence: recommendations are essential to informed decision making. *BMJ*. 2013 Dec 19;*347*:f7600.

Stiggelbout AM, Van der Weijden T, DeWit MPT, et al. Shared decision making: really putting patients at the centre of healthcare. *BMJ*. 2012;*344*;e256.

Venkatesh AK, Schuur JD. A "top five" list for emergency medicine: a policy and research agenda for stewardship to improve the value of emergency care. *Am J Emerg Med*. 2013 Oct;*31*(10):1520–1524.

17 "12/10" Abdominal Pain

Chadd K. Kraus

A 36-year-old female presents to the emergency department (ED) of a small, community hospital with sharp, stabbing, "12/10" lower abdominal and pelvic pain with nausea, but no fever, vomiting, or diarrhea. Chart review reveals an allergy to nonsteroidal anti-inflammatory drugs (NSAIDs), a history of chronic abdominal pain, depression, two cesarean sections, an appendectomy, ovarian cysts, and multiple ED visits with documented concern for "drug-seeking behavior." The chart shows the patient had computed tomography (CT) of the abdomen and pelvis 2 weeks ago and a pelvic ultrasound 3 weeks ago, both of which showed no etiologies for her symptoms.

Vital signs are heart rate 105 beats per minute, blood pressure 118/79 mm Hg, respiratory rate 18 breaths per minute, and temperature 98.8°F. When you enter the room, the patient writhes in pain, screaming, "My stomach hurts!" On examination, she appears to be in pain, but has diffuse, minimal pain to palpation—inconsistent with her subjective report of pain. Her examination is otherwise unremarkable. You try to elicit more history, and she refuses to answer, saying, "I need something for this pain, RIGHT NOW!"

What do you do now?

DRUG-SEEKING BEHAVIOR

Pain is the most common reason for presentation to the ED. Treating pain and eliciting the etiology of pain are fundamental responsibilities of emergency physicians. For most patients presenting to the ED, pain is a symptom of an underlying injury or illness. In a small subset of patients, pain is the result of a more complex constellation that could include an acute injury or illness or a manifestation of drug addiction and dependence. Frequently termed *drug-seeking behavior*, presentations of pain in patients with a history of drug misuse or drug addiction and dependence that are unrelated to an acute injury or illness can pose an ethical dilemma for emergency physicians. On one hand, emergency physicians have a duty, dictated by the ethical principle of beneficence, to treat patients with respect and dignity within the context of the patient-physician compact. The appropriate and adequate treatment of pain in the ED is a duty of the emergency physician within the patient-physician relationship. On the other hand, providing medications to a patient in the acute setting of the ED that might exacerbate the underlying illness of addiction and dependence can be harmful to that particular patient. The emergency physician's autonomy is to make treatment decisions based on a clinical judgment about what will be beneficial or harmful to the patient. However, clinical judgment can be interrupted by feelings of frustration, resentment, or distrust experienced by the emergency physician when faced with a patient suspected of, or with a history of, drug-seeking behavior who presents with a complaint of pain, particularly after repeated ED visits or with a discordant history and examination.

Further complicating this dilemma is the difficulty in accurately identifying patients with drug-seeking behavior, particularly with the heightened attention to drug abuse in the current opioid epidemic. Patients with drug-seeking behavior historically have high rates of ED utilization. Although frequently described in the literature and anecdotally among physicians, "classic" drug-seeking behaviors such as complaining of headache, back, or dental pain; losing prescriptions; or asking for medications by name only occur with low-to-moderate frequency. Nevertheless, some clinical factors have been associated with drug-seeking behavior in ED patients: reported allergies to nonnarcotic medications; reported stolen medications; requesting medications by name; requesting intravenous opioids; multiple ED visits for the same complaints; reporting 10 out of 10 pain; suspicious history; symptoms out of proportion to examination results; no primary care physician reported by patient.

CASE RESOLUTION

It is crucial to convey to the patient a sincere desire to control her pain and to evaluate her symptoms while at the same time balancing the need to avoid or minimize harm (i.e., the principle of nonmaleficence or, to "do no harm"). The physician should express the nonjudgmental concern to the patient about the risks of drug abuse and share available resources for addiction and dependence treatment. The equilibrium between addressing a patient's pain and minimizing harm hinges on an appropriate, objective history, examination, and diagnostic evaluation.

In this case, the emergency physician should use adequate and evidence-based pain management strategies, which may or may not include opioids, while evaluating the patient for an acute etiology of her symptoms, such as cholecystitis. Particularly in cases where medication misuse and abuse are a concern, the emergency physician should avoid personalizing the situation and employ an objective approach to exclude acute etiologies for the patient's symptoms. The conversation with the patient should focus on the acute presentation and if necessary express general concern about the patient's safety in the context of drug use. Example language might include, "I am concerned about a serious cause of your symptoms. While we evaluate you further in the emergency department, we will give you medications to help with your pain. We also are obligated to balance controlling your pain and maintaining safety, as pain medications can be dangerous."

If the ED evaluation does not reveal an acute etiology, the emergency physician should follow applicable laws and professional society guidelines regarding the use of opioids for this patient after the ED visit to determine any additional pain management strategies. Importantly, the decision to prescribe any outpatient opioids at the time of discharge from the ED should be evidence based and should be made in the context of the patient's overall pain management strategy (e.g., is she being followed by a pain management specialist, or should such a referral be initiated in the ED?).

The use of objective tools, such as a prescription drug monitoring program (PDMP) database might help identify patients at high risk for drug seeking. PDMP use should adhere to general ethical principles and should be undertaken with an understanding of the limitations of such tools. In the case presented here, the emergency physician must develop and consider differential diagnoses for this patient's symptoms and offer testing appropriate to evaluate for those diagnoses based on clinical judgment. Emergent etiologies for the patient's pain must be excluded and might require diagnostic testing, such as laboratory or imaging studies. The emergency physician should not assume that the patient has no injury or illness and is simply drug seeking. Nonnarcotic, nonpharmacologic, or opioids or other analgesics might be the appropriate treatment for a patient with a history of drug-seeking behavior, addiction, or dependence depending on the clinical situation.

KEY POINTS TO REMEMBER

- Treating pain and eliciting the etiology of pain are fundamental responsibilities of emergency physicians.
- Historical features alone might be inadequate or inaccurate in discerning if the patient is drug seeking.
- It is crucial to convey to the patient a sincere desire to control her pain and to evaluate her symptoms while at the same time balancing the need to avoid harm.
- Analgesia, including opioids, might be appropriate for patients who are exhibiting drug-seeking behavior and is dependent on the clinical situation.

Suggested Reading

American College of Emergency Physicians (ACEP). Policy statement: electronic prescription drug monitoring programs. Approved January 2017. Available at: https://www.acep.org/globalassets/new-pdfs/policy-statements/electronic-prescription-drug-monitoring-programs.pdf. Accessed September 16, 2019.

American College of Emergency Physicians (ACEP). Policy statement: optimizing the treatment of acute pain in the ED. Approved April 2017. Available at: https://www.

acep.org/globalassets/new-pdfs/policy-statements/optimizing-the-treatment-of-acute-pain-in-the-ed.pdf. Accessed September 16, 2019.

Cantrill SV, Brown MD, Carlisle RJ, et al. Clinical policy: critical issues in the prescribing of opioids for adult patients in the emergency department. *Ann Emerg Med*. 2012;*60*(4):499–525.

Elder JW, DePalma G, Pines JM. Optimal implementation of prescription drug monitoring programs in the emergency department. *West J Emerg Med*. 2018;*19*(2):387–391.

Grover CA, Close RJ, Wiele ED, et al. Quantifying drug-seeking behavior: a case control study. *J Emerg Med*. 2012;*42*(1):15–21.

Grover CA, Elder JW, Close RJH, Curry SM. How frequently are "classic" drug-seeking behaviors used by drug-seeking patients in the emergency department? *West J Emerg Med*. 2012;*13*(5):416–421.

Marco CA, Venkat A, Baker EF, et al. Prescription drug monitoring programs: ethical issues in the emergency department. *Ann Emerg Med*. 2016;*68*(5):589–598.

Weiner SG, Griggs CA, Langlois BK, et al. Characteristics of emergency department "doctor shoppers." *J Emerg Med*. 2015;*48*(4):424–431.

Weiner SG, Griggs CA, Mitchell PM, et al. Clinical impression versus prescription drug monitoring program criteria in the assessment of drug-seeking behavior in the emergency department. *Ann Emerg Med*. 2013;*62*:281–289.

Zechnich AD, Hedges JR. Community-wide emergency department visits by patients suspected of drug-seeking behavior. *Acad Emerg Med*. 1996;*3*(4):312–317.

18 Fear and Loathing in the ED

Thomas E. Robey and Jay M. Brenner

A 29-year-old man arrives to the emergency department
(ED) by private vehicle complaining of flu-like symptoms.
After several hours in the waiting room, he is moved to
the treatment area. After intake, the nurse exits the room
as you review his chart. In the last 6 months, he was
seen nine times at your hospital for a range of problems,
including abscesses, psychosis, heroin overdose, and upper
respiratory infections. When you enter the room, you notice
an anxious, disheveled man answering clinical history
questions with one or two word sentences. You extract
complaints of body aches, nausea, diarrhea, and cold sweats
for about 1 day. Though he is guarded about his symptoms,
he freely criticizes your waiting room, the long wait, and
the prejudice he feels has been applied to him. When his
nurse performs the nasopharyngeal swab for influenza, he
strikes her arm and knocks her back to the wall. You bolt to
the room while he berates her, saying, "All you have to do is
give me some oxys."

What do you do now?

INTOXICATION AND SUBSTANCE ABUSE

Opiate use disorder (OUD) has reached epidemic proportion. In 2017, there were 2.4 million Americans addicted to heroin or prescription opiates, and 47,000 people died as the result of opiate overdose. Despite an annual economic burden of $78.5 billion, access to medical and mental health treatment remains a challenge for patients with OUD. Combining social stigma of drug abuse with the physical dependence on the drug and individual economic consequences of drug use makes the ED the front line for evaluation and treatment of many direct consequences of OUD, namely overdose, withdrawal, and psychosis from polysubstance use; and indirect consequences of drug use, including skin infections, injuries, and environmental exposure.

This case highlights the nexus of opiate withdrawal with workplace violence and requires immediate decisions by the physician to protect the patient and staff. Without the time to conduct an ethical analysis, the physician must act justly while keeping the patient's interest in mind. Prior to the violent outburst, it may not have been immediately apparent that the opiate-dependent patient presenting with flu-like symptoms (as with previous ED use for viral syndromes) was actually in severe withdrawal, but when staff are threatened, a temporizing measure to keep all parties safe is indicated. Physical restraints applied by a trained security team will minimize patient injury and should be applied as soon as possible. Unlike in organic psychosis, impulsive behaviors can be transient in opiate withdrawal; long-acting chemical restraints may not be needed and could delay appropriate treatment.

With the intent of protecting all parties, the initial act of placing the patient in restraints not only is justified by quality standards to protect the staff and patient, but also is beneficent and nonmaleficent at that time. This seemingly contradicts patient autonomy. When the outburst is viewed as an impulsive behavior in the context of the patient's attempt to quit, the patient's intent becomes less clear. A spot determination of capacity is needed in order to fully confer autonomous decision-making ability to the intoxicated patient. Many patients in this situation may neither possess the ability to understand the medical situation nor demonstrate rational decision-making with regard to a treatment decision. In some cases, autonomy may be further suspended. Involuntary treatment for drug or alcohol abuse is an option in 37 states. Variable requirements for commitment mesh with underresourced systems, but in general, laws enable physicians to involuntarily detain patients who demonstrate grave disability due to dependence on drugs or alcohol using a similar mechanism for suicidal and psychotic patients.

CASE RESOLUTION

When the possibility appears that his physical and behavioral symptoms are secondary to withdrawal, the provider has an opening to build rapport with the patient. "I know I just put you in restraints, but I'm getting the sense that it's your craving for heroin that controlled your actions. How long has it been since your last use?" will acknowledge your patient's personal struggle with opiates. Perhaps he has been trying to quit, but could not handle the stress of physiologic withdrawal. He did come to the ED for help. Meeting him where he is, which means treating him with dignity and respect, will help shed the stigma and bias you may unconsciously carry into the room. Furthermore, though prescription-monitoring programs can reduce controlled substance prescription rates, these and other internal lists—including care plans—of frequent utilizers have the potential to interfere with rapport or breach ethical and professional standards by violating trust or confidentiality when used separate from prescription decisions.

Once you establish rapport, clinical therapeutics should be used to treat the opiate withdrawal symptoms. Clonidine, antiemetics, antidiarrheals, and benzodiazepines are the most common agents dispensed and prescribed. As experience with partial mu-receptor agonists expands, induction for medication-assisted therapy (MAT) using buprenorphine or methadone has been implemented in the ED. Such programs have reduced opiate misuse and boosted compliance with drug treatment programs. As relationships between EDs and local treatment centers develop, it is incumbent on emergency providers to offer this option to help opiate-dependent individuals have the opportunity to escape their addiction. Induction and 3 days of initial treatment does not require a Drug Enforcement Administration (DEA) waiver. Beginning the process of addiction treatment is the best outcome for this patient.

Suggested Reading

Bao Y, Pan Y, Taylor A, et al. Prescription drug monitoring programs are associated with sustained reductions in opioid prescribing by physicians. *Health Aff (Millwood)*. 2016 Jun 1;*35*(6):1045–1051.

Brenner JM, Hashmi J. The difficult patient. In: Marco C, Schears R (eds.), *Ethical Dilemmas in Emergency Medicine*. New York: Cambridge University Press; 2015: Chap. 10.

CDC/NCHS, National Vital Statistics System, Mortality. CDC WONDER. Atlanta, GA: US Department of Health and Human Services, CDC; 2018. https://wonder.cdc.gov. Accessed March 21, 2019.

Center for Behavioral Health Statistics and Quality (CBHSQ). *2017 National Survey on Drug Use and Health: Detailed Tables*. Rockville, MD: Substance Abuse and Mental Health Services Administration; 2018.

D'Onofrio G, O'Connor PG, Pantalon MV, et al. Emergency department-initiated buprenorphine/naloxone treatment for opioid dependence: a randomized clinical trial. *JAMA*. 2015 Apr 28;*313*(16):1636–1644.

Florence CS, Zhou C, Luo F, et al. The economic burden of prescription opioid overdose, abuse, and dependence in the United States. *Med Care*. 2016;*54*(10):901–906.

Geiderman JM. Keeping lists and naming names: habitual patient files for suspected nontherapeutic drug-seeking patients. *Ann Emerg Med*. 2003;*42*:873–881.

Joint Commission on Accreditation of Healthcare Organizations (JCAHO). Standards PC.03.05.01 through PC.03.05.19. https://www.jointcommission.org/assets. Accessed March 14, 2019.

Kreisman E, Gang M, Goldfrank LR. The interface: ethical decision making, medical toxicology, and emergency medicine. *Emerg Med Clin N Am*. 2006;*24*:769–784.

Levinson I, Galynker II, Rosenthal RN. Methadone withdrawal psychosis. *J Clin Psychiatry*. 1995 Feb;*56*(2):73–76.

Revised Code of Washington Chapter 71.05: Involuntary Treatment Act ("Ricky's Law"). https://apps.leg.wa.gov/rcw/default.aspx?cite=71.05. Accessed March 24, 2019.

19 Everyday J.

Chadd K. Kraus

"J." is a middle-aged man who seeks care in his local emergency department (ED) two or three times per week. He has multiple health problems, including diabetes mellitus (DM), coronary artery disease (CAD), chronic obstructive pulmonary disease (COPD), hypertension (HTN), and chronic back pain due to an old work injury. His visits are usually for acute exacerbations of these conditions. When J. presents to the ED, staff lament another "unnecessary visit by this frequent flier" and have given him the nickname, "Everyday J." In an attempt to reduce his ED utilization, the health system has put in place multiple social and hospital case management services assisting home care, medication management, and care coordination.

J. presents to your ED with chest pain, dyspnea, and "not feeling right." He had provocative testing 3 months ago that showed stable CAD. His chest x-ray, laboratory tests, and electrocardiogram (ECG) are all reassuring, without evidence of an acute etiology. You discuss the test results with J., and he reports to you that he is also having difficulty walking due to worsening back pain over the past day.

What do you do now?

EMERGENCY DEPARTMENT SUPERUSERS

Commonly defined as having greater than four ED visits in a year, patients who are frequent users of the ED make up an estimated 3.5% to 10% of all ED visits and have been reported to account for nearly a third of all ED use. Patients who are frequent users of the ED are often referred to as "superusers" or "frequent fliers" and can be a source of frustration to ED staff and a source of concern surrounding disproportionate resource utilization among health systems and third-party payers.

There are multiple misconceptions surrounding frequent ED users. Some of these include a lack of access to primary care and ED visits for nonemergent symptoms or conditions. Contrary to these myths, patients with the highest ED utilization are a heterogeneous group. Some themes have emerged in the literature, including that these patients are in overall poorer health than patients who use the ED less and they do not use the ED as a substitute for outpatient primary care. Frequent ED users have higher mortality, higher hospital admission rates, and higher use of all health care services, both specialty and primary care, compared to other patients using the ED. These patients have similar linkages to outpatient care in comparison to patients who use the ED less frequently. They are more likely to be homeless and are more likely to be publicly insured (e.g., Medicare or Medicaid). Among frequent users of emergency medical services (EMS), there is a predominance of male gender and a high burden of alcohol use. Reducing frequent ED use has been a priority for hospitals, health systems, payers, and governments, although many of these programs have been controversial and variable in impact, with no specific intervention emerging as superior.

CASE RESOLUTION

J. is at high risk for serious pathology given his complex medical history. The emergency physician must balance the potential for acute medical conditions in J. with an appreciation and concern for the need for stewardship in the prudent application of finite resources in the ED. J. should have the autonomy to access ED evaluation and care if he believes he has a medical emergency. This principle has been codified into both federal and many state laws protecting the "prudent layperson standard." He should not be coerced not to seek ED care if he believes he has an emergent condition. The emergency physician must work to communicate effectively with J. regarding the necessity and harms of certain diagnostic tests and treatments, while also appreciating the risks of acute decompensation of his many medical conditions. In this case, J. is less likely to have a cardiac or pulmonary etiology for his presenting symptoms; however, the emergency physician must also give adequate consideration, via history and examination, to potential serious etiologies of low back pain in J.

The emergency physician should reevaluate J. to determine if his back pain is an acute issue. If he has signs of neurologic deficit or other red flag signs or symptoms, the emergency physician should order appropriate diagnostic testing, including laboratory tests and imaging if warranted, and if necessary, consult a specialist or arrange transfer to a higher level of care where specialist evaluation is available. Based on his past medical history, including back injuries, J. could have a serious cause of his back pain, including infection or cord compression. The emergency physician is obligated to address a patient's symptoms to exclude an emergent or life-, limb-, or sight-threatening etiology. Additionally, the emergency physician should address, in an empathetic manner, the concerns surrounding J's frequent use of the ED. The emergency physician might inquire, "We are concerned that you come to the ED frequently because we aren't addressing your needs. Do you have other concerns, like housing or family/friends, outside of your health that bring you to the ED? Do you feel that you are receiving the care that you need to meet your medical issues, or is there another resource that we might be able to arrange for you?" The emergency physician could also request that a case manager, social worker, or other available resource be included in J's care during this ED visit to confirm that previously established care management plans are being adequately implemented and accessed.

KEY POINTS TO REMEMBER

· Patients with the highest ED utilization are in overall poorer health than patients who use the ED less.

- Frequent users generally do not use the ED as a substitute for outpatient primary care.
- Reducing frequent ED use has been a priority for hospitals, health systems, payers, and governments, although many of these programs have been controversial and variable in impact.
- Patients should not be coerced to avoid ED care.
- Serious etiologies for symptoms in frequent users must be considered.

Suggested Reading

Billings J, Raven MC. Dispelling an urban legend: frequent emergency department users have substantial burden of disease. *Health Aff.* 2013;*32*(12):2099–2108.

Doran KM, Raven MC, Rosenheck RA. What drives frequent emergency department use in an integrated health system? National data from the Veterans Health Administration. *Ann Emerg Med.* 2013;*6*(2):151–159.

Doupe MB, Palatnick W, Day S, et al. Frequent users of emergency departments: developing standard definitions and defining prominent risk factors. *Ann Emerg Med.* 2012;*60*(1):24–32.

Grover CA, Crawford E, Close RJH, The efficacy of case management on emergency department frequent users: an eight-year observational study. *J Emerg Med.* 2016;*51*(5):595–604.

Hall MK, Raven MC, Hall J, et al. EMS-STARS: Emergency medical services "superuser" transport associations: an adult retrospective study. *Prehosp Emerg Care.* 2015;*19*:61–67.

Hunt KA, Weber EJ, Showstack JA, et al. Characteristics of frequent users of emergency departments. *Ann Emerg Med.* 2006;*48*(1):1–8.

Ku BS, Fields JM, Santana A, et al. The urban homeless: super-users of the emergency department. *Popul Health Manag.* 2014;*17*:366–371.

LaCalle E, Rabin E. Frequent users of emergency departments: the myths, the data, and the policy implications. *Ann Emerg Med.* 2010;*56*(1):42–48.

Locker TE, Baston S, Mason SM. et al. Defining frequent use of an urban emergency department. *Emerg Med J.* 2007;*24*:398–401.

Moe J, Kirkland S, Ospina MB, et al. Mortality, admission rates and outpatient use among frequent users of emergency departments: a systematic review. *Emerg Med J.* 2016;*33*(3):230–236.

Phillips GA, Brophy DS, Weiland TJ, et al. The effect of multidisciplinary case management on selected outcomes for frequent attenders at an emergency department. *Med J Aust.* 2006;*184*(12):602–606.

Sun BC, Burstin HR, Brennan TA. Predictors and outcomes of frequent emergency
  department users. *Acad Emerg Med.* 2003;*10*(4):320–328.

Van den Heede K, Van de Voorde C. Interventions to reduce emergency department
  utilization: a review of reviews. *Health Policy.* 2016;*120*(12):1337–1349.

Zuckerman S, Shen YC. Characteristics of occasional and frequent emergency
  department users: do insurance coverage and access to care matter? *Med Care.*
  2004;*42*(2):176–182.

20 "I Want a Baby, But Not With Him"

Simiao Li-Sauerwine and
Diane L. Gorgas

A 27-year-old woman presents to the emergency department (ED) requesting emergency contraception. She reports having consensual unprotected intercourse 2 days ago. She reveals that she is hoping to have a child with her partner, but "messed up and was with this other guy—I want to have a baby, but not with him." She denies trauma, history of sexually transmitted infections (STIs), or other pregnancies. She has no vaginal bleeding and reports scant discharge. Her last menstrual period was 3 weeks ago. She endorses no medical illnesses and takes no medications. Physical examination reveals a pleasant, moderately obese woman with a body mass index (BMI) of 32. Her abdominal and pelvic examinations are benign. The remainder of her examination is normal. You contact your clinical pharmacist for recommendations on the most effective oral emergency contraceptive given the patient's higher BMI, but the response from your pharmacist is, "She had consensual sex; this wasn't rape. Shouldn't she live with her decision. . . . Does she really need emergency contraception?"

What do you do now?

EMERGENCY CONTRACEPTION IN THE
EMERGENCY DEPARTMENT

In this case, a nulligravid young woman presents to the ED requesting emergency contraception after consensual intercourse. This case is complicated by the fact that she currently desires to become pregnant, but not with this partner. She has no contraindications to emergency contraception, and she is within the time window when it would likely be effective; however, your clinical pharmacist questions its necessity based on personal moral grounds.

In considering provision of emergency contraception, it's important to note that a broad range of national organizations, such as the Centers for Disease Control and Prevention, the American College of Emergency Physicians, and the American College of Obstetricians and Gynecologists, support the provision of emergency contraception. Further, these organizations recommend that emergency contraception should be recommended to *all* women who have had unprotected or inadequately protected intercourse and who do not desire pregnancy. There are no conditions which have been identified in which the risk of emergency contraception is outweighed by the benefits it offers, including in cases of previous ectopic pregnancy, cardiovascular disease, migraines, liver disease, or in women who are breastfeeding.

While the emergency department isn't the ideal setting for patients to seek emergency contraception, it is important to realize that an emergency physician denying a patient's request can result in a delay in care which might cause them to be outside of the effective treatment window. While in an optimal situation, patients would be able to obtain emergency contraception from a primary care provider, gynecologist, or directly from a pharmacy, emergency physicians should not refuse to provide emergency contraception based on the setting of the request. The role of emergency physicians is to serve as a safety net for those unable to reach other resources. It is also important to consider that deferring provision of emergency contraception to outpatient providers imposes a higher burden of effort to those who are socioeconomically disadvantaged and can result in discriminatory prescribing with respect to who has access to emergency contraception in a timely manner.

There is a disparity in the likelihood of a provider to offer emergency contraception based on the circumstances surrounding an instance of unprotected intercourse. Providers are far more likely to offer emergency contraception in cases of sexual assault compared to consensual intercourse. Among ED physicians and nurses, a study regarding adolescent patients seeking emergency contraception found that there exists a punitive attitude—that unintended pregnancy is the price to pay for "irresponsible behavior." Some providers also revealed judgments based on patients' perceived potential (i.e., an adolescent who is college bound vs. someone who did not complete high school). Although it can be frustrating to providers when patients fail to seek preventive measures, it is unethical for providers to withhold treatment due to prior patient nonadherence to ideal practices or social standing. Other barriers cited include provider lack of familiarity with provision of emergency contraception, including appropriate prescribing practices, side effects, and contraindications. It is incumbent on emergency physicians to be appropriately educated regarding the provision of emergency contraception as it is within their scope of practice.

CASE RESOLUTION

Conscientious objection has been cited by providers who are unwilling to participate in the provision of emergency contraception. Some physicians and ancillary staff may refuse to provide emergency contraception because they feel that provision of contraception is immoral. In this situation, the interests of providers and patients are at odds. In considering provision of emergency contraception as viewed through the principles of autonomy, nonmaleficence, and beneficence, all factors weigh in favor of the patient. With respect to autonomy, individuals must have access to necessary information in order to make informed health care choices; to respect autonomy, providers must ensure that a patient's decision is informed and voluntary. Although providers have a right to their beliefs, these beliefs cannot infringe on the health and safety of others. It is unethical for the provider to withhold information pertaining to a patient's medical care, and it is his or her duty to provide necessary information. While it is possible to refer the patient to a willing provider, efficacy of emergency contraception is time sensitive, and delays in care will result in a less effective or ineffective medication.

Regarding nonmaleficence, a provider's refusal to provide emergency contraception inflicts harm on the patient by exposing her to the risks of an unintended pregnancy. Adherence to nonmaleficence includes provision of "due care"; in the case of unprotected intercourse, standard of care as defined by professional medical organizations includes provision of emergency contraception. Of note, this recommendation does not differentiate between consensual intercourse and sexual assault. Finally, the principle of beneficence obligates providers to act in the benefit of the patient, rather than to simply refrain from doing harm. In plain terms, providers must act to benefit the patient and in accordance with the standard of care, rather than abstaining due to personal convictions.

KEY POINTS TO REMEMBER

- Emergency contraception should be offered to *all* women who have unprotected intercourse who do not desire pregnancy.
- There are no contraindications to emergency contraception based on underlying medical condition.
- It is the duty of providers to seek education regarding appropriate prescribing practices for emergency contraception.
- Conscientious objection to provision of emergency contraception by providers is not supported by the ethical principles of autonomy, nonmaleficence, or beneficence.

Suggested Reading

Abbott J, Feldhaus KM, Houry D, Lowenstein SR. (2004). Emergency contraception: what do our patients know? *Ann Emerg Med.* *43*(3):376–381. doi:https://www.annemergmed.com/article/S0196-0644(03)01120-X/fulltext

American College of Obstetricians and Gynecologists. (2015). *Emergency Contraception. Practice Bulletin: Clinical Management Guidelines for Obstetrician-Gynecologists; Number 152.* Washington, DC: American College of Obstetricians and Gynecologists.

Card RF. Conscientious objection and emergency contraception. *Am J Bioethics.* 2007;7(6):8–14. doi:10.1080/15265160701347239

Keshavarz R, Merchant RC, McGreal J. Emergency contraception provision: a survey of emergency department practitioners. *Acad Emerg Med*. 2002;9(1):69–74.

Miller MK, Plantz DM, Dowd MD, et al. Pediatric emergency health care providers' knowledge, attitudes, and experiences regarding emergency contraception. *Acad Emerg Med*. 2011;18(6):605–612. doi:10.1111/j.1553-2712.2011.01079.x

Thilo RC. Barriers and biases: ethical considerations for providing emergency contraception to adolescents in the emergency department. *Virtual Mentor*. 2012;14(2):121–125. doi:10.1001/virtualmentor.2012.14.2.jdsc1-1202

Weisberg E, Fraser IS. Emergency contraception. *Int J Gyn Obst*. 2009;106:160–163. doi:10.1016/j.ijgo.2009.03.031

21 Risky Behavior

Catherine A. Marco

A 28-year-old woman presents to the emergency department (ED) following unprotected sex with a partner previously unknown to her. She volunteers that she regularly engages in prostitution. She is worried that she may get HIV from this person. She is requesting HIV testing and postexposure prophylaxis (PEP). She also is requesting that the police find the individual for mandated HIV testing. She had multiple, previous, similar encounters and was treated with 28 days of PEP 6 months previously.

What do you do now?

RISKS AND BENEFITS OF POSTEXPOSURE PROPHYLAXIS

HIV exposure may result in seroconversion, through either occupational or nonoccupational exposure. Nonoccupational exposure typically includes sexual contact or exposure to infected blood or body fluids. Worldwide, intercourse is the most common transmission route. In the United States, male-to-male sexual contact and injection drug use are common routes of transmission.

Postexposure prophylaxis with antiretroviral therapy (ART) can reduce the risk of HIV transmission. It is estimated that PEP can prevent 90% of potential transmissions. This is dependent on patient compliance, timing of initiation of therapy, and risk. The decision to administer PEP should be based on risk of HIV acquisition; time elapsed after exposure, and potential for drug toxicity. Nonoccupational PEP (nPEP) should be offered to patients with a moderate-to-high risk of exposure, and a source patient with known HIV infection or high risk of HIV should be considered for PEP. Ideally, PEP must be started within 72 hours of exposure. PEP is not recommended if the risk of transmission is low or if the source patient is HIV negative. Typically, a three-drug regimen for a 28-day course is recommended. PEP therapy has a significant risk of adverse reactions, including gastrointestinal upset, renal toxicity, hepatotoxicity, neuropathy, pancreatitis, lactic acidosis syndrome, rash, headache, and others. Decisions should be made using shared decision-making with the patient, to include discussions regarding risks and benefits, and consultation with infectious disease or the National Clinician's Postexposure Prophylaxis Hotline.

Patient education and counseling are important components of ART initiation. Patients should be counseled to avoid pregnancy and to practice sexual abstinence or condom use and to refrain from donating blood, organs, tissue, or semen for 12 months.

Preexposure prophylaxis (PrPEP) should be considered for patients who frequently engage in high-risk behaviors. PrPEP can reduce the risk of HIV transmission by greater than 90%. PrPEP should be considered for patients who have received more than one course of nPEP in the past year. Patients engaging in high-risk behaviors should also be tested for sexually transmitted infection, such as syphilis, gonorrhea, or chlamydia; and for hepatitis B and C infection. PrPEP requires access to prescription medication, outpatient follow-up, and patient adherence to a daily medication regimen. The Centers for Disease Control and Prevention (CDC) estimates that only a minority of patients eligible for PrPEP use actually used PrPEP.

TESTING OF PATIENT AND SOURCE

Testing of the exposed person is recommended. PEP may be administered pending results to ensure timely administration. Testing of the source patient is ideal if the patient is willing and available. If the source patient can be identified, informed consent should be obtained prior to HIV testing.

State laws vary regarding HIV testing. Many states have laws that permit unconsented HIV testing of source patients following an occupational exposure to a health care provider. Some states require a court order for unconsented HIV testing. State laws vary regarding the procedures for unconsented testing, including authorization, documentation, and results reporting.

Many states have laws requiring persons who are aware of HIV infection to disclose their status to sexual partners. Legal advice regarding charges against state law is beyond the scope of the ED, and patients should be referred to legal counsel.

ETHICAL CONSIDERATIONS

Autonomy

Respect for patient autonomy refers to respect for an individual's right to make medical decisions about his or her own body. Providers should respect the right of patients to make medical decisions that reflect their own goals and values. Decisions should be based on clear and accurate information, and should be free of coercion. Regarding nPEP and PrPEP, the individual patient should participate in an assessment of the risks and benefits and decision to administer these medications. Testing of the source patient brings to light the question of autonomy and ability to consent for this patient. These two duties may conflict, for example, if an exposed person wishes the source patient to be tested who declines testing.

Beneficence

Beneficence, the obligation to act in the best interest of patients, applies to this decision. The provider has a duty to do good, or to promote the patient's welfare. In general, PEP is an effective medication regimen. However, the risk of adverse reactions is significant and should be discussed with the patient prior to the decision to administer PEP. The best possible treatment should be offered without judgment of the patient's lifestyle choices.

Nonmaleficence

Nonmaleficence, the obligation to not inflict harm intentionally, has application in this case. Nonmaleficence often references the phrase *primum non nocere* ("first, do no harm"). This principle mandates that the provider should avoid any action that would intentionally harm the patient. Some make the ethical argument that administration of PEP or PrPEP may validate the immoral or risky behavior. However, most agree that a medically efficacious treatment should be administered without judgment of the patient's future risk for continued behavior. Similar arguments have been made for other treatments for patients exhibiting risky behavior, such as needle exchange programs, postcoital contraception, or naloxone for home treatment of opioid overdose. The potential for risky behavior should be recognized and the patient should be counseled about the risk for acquiring other sexually transmitted infections or conditions.

Justice

Justice, the duty of fairness in processes and distribution of benefits, applies to this case. Justice includes three categories: distribution of scarce resources, respect for patient's rights, and respect for morally acceptable laws. Although PEP therapy is expensive, evidence suggests that it is cost effective in preventing disease transmission. Some would argue that the high cost could be better spent on prevention and education. Although we support these measures, in general, the high cost of treatment should not influence the care of an individual patient if proven to be efficacious.

Patient Education

Risky sexual behavior is associated with numerous conditions, including sexually transmitted diseases and mental health disorders. Risky sexual behavior leads to the majority of HIV transmission in the United States. Patients should be counseled regarding risks and benefits of antiretroviral therapy, as well as risks of unprotected sex. Although counseling may be initiated in the ED, time often does not allow for adequate lifestyle counseling. Follow-up resources should be provided with infectious disease, primary care, and social services.

FUTURE DIRECTIONS

Comprehensive and consistent treatment of patients who would benefit from nPEP and PrPEP should be a goal of treatment. This may be facilitated by the use of institutional and national clinical guidelines, training curricula, and improved communication with patients to assist in shared decision-making for the best options to provide ideal medical care in harmony with individual patient goals and values. Future medical research may further elucidate the efficacy of nPEP and PrPEP, as well as alternative drug regimens with potentially lower potential for adverse effects.

CASE RESOLUTION

This patient demonstrates repeated risky sexual behavior. Other psychosocial factors should be investigated, such as the possibility of abuse, drug use, mental health conditions, and capacity. She should be counseled on the importance of safe sexual practices. She should be assessed for the risk of exposure, and the HIV status of the source patient should be considered, if known. If unknown, the patient may be requested to undergo HIV testing. In some states, unconsented HIV testing may be legally permissible. This patient and the physician should, through shared decision-making, make the best decision regarding nPEP and possible referral for PrPEP. You explain that the police do not investigate possible HIV exposures, but the health department will perform contact tracing. The patient should be counseled regarding the importance of compliance with prescribed medications and should be referred to primary care, infectious disease, and if indicated, social services for counseling and further recommendations.

· Postexposure prophylaxis is effective in reducing postexposure HIV seroconversion.

· Postexposure prophylaxis should be initiated within 72 hours of exposure.

· Persons who demonstrate high-risk exposure may benefit from preexposure prophylaxis.

· Persons who engage in risky sexual behavior should be counseled about safe sexual practices.

Suggested Reading

Brawner BM, Alexander KA, Fannin EF, et al. The role of sexual health professionals in developing a shared concept of risky sexual behavior as it relates to HIV transmission. *Public Health Nurs*. 2016 Mar–Apr;*33*(2):139–150.

Centers for Disease Control and Prevention. HIV and STD criminal laws. Available at: https://www.cdc.gov/hiv/policies/law/states/exposure.html. Accessed February 22, 2019.

Centers for Disease Control and Prevention. HIV Surveillance Report, 2017, vol. *29*. Available at: https://www.cdc.gov/hiv/pdf/library/reports/surveillance/cdc-hiv-surveillance-report-2017-vol-29.pdf. Accessed February 11, 2019.

Centers for Disease Control and Prevention. Updated guidelines for antiretroviral postexposure prophylaxis after sexual, injection drug use, or other nonoccupational exposure to HIV—United States. 2016. Available at: https://www.cdc.gov/mmwR/preview/mmwrhtml/rr5402a1.htm. Accessed February 2, 2019.

Clinician Consultation Center. PEP: Post-exposure prophylaxis. Available at: http://nccc.ucsf.edu/clinician-consultation/pep-post-exposure-prophylaxis/. Accessed February 11, 2019.

Cowan E, Macklin R: Unconsented HIV testing in cases of occupational exposure: ethics, law, and policy. *Acad Emerg Med*. 2012 October;*19*(10):1181–1187.

Gisondi MA. Post-exposure prophylaxis for HIV following possible sexual transmission: an ethical evaluation. *Cambridge Q Healthc Ethics*. 2000;9:411–417.

Maclean JC, Xu H, French MT, et al. Mental health and risky sexual behaviors: evidence from *DSM-IV* Axis II disorders. *J Ment Health Policy Econ*. 2013 Dec;*16*(4):187–208.

Marcus JL, Katz KA, Krakower DS, et al. Risk compensation and clinical decision making—the case of HIV preexposure prophylaxis. *N Engl J Med*. 2019 Feb 7;*380*(6):510–512.

Pinkerton SD, Martin JN, Roland WE, et al. Cost-effectiveness of postexposure prophylaxis after sexual or injection-drug exposure to human immunodeficiency virus. *Arch Intern Med*. 2004;*164*:46–54.

Ross DA. Behavioural interventions to reduce HIV risk: what works? *AIDS*. 2010 Oct;*24*(suppl 4):S4–S14.

Seidner MJ, Tumarkin E, Bogoch IIL. HIV post-exposure prophylaxis (PEP). *BMJ*. 2018;*363*:k4928.

Sugarman J, Mayer KH. Ethics and pre-exposure prophylaxis for HIV-infection. *J Acquir Immune Defic Syndr*. 2013 July;*63*(0 2):S135–S139.

UNAIDS Gap Report 2014. Available at: https://www.unaids.org/en/resources/documents/2014/20140716_UNAIDS_gap_report. Accessed February 2, 2020.

Walzer AS, Van Manen KL, Ryan CS. Other- versus self-focus and risky health behavior: the case of HIV/AIDS. *Psychol Health Med*. 2016 Oct;*21*(7):902–907.

22 Little Secrets, Big Lies

Simiao Li-Sauerwine and
Diane L. Gorgas

A 12-year-old male presents to the emergency department
with his parents. He has had progressive fatigue and
intermittent fevers over the past several weeks. They have
recently moved to the area from out of state and have not
yet established care with a primary care physician. The boy
has a history of mild asthma for which he takes an inhaler.
He has no other significant medical history and takes no
other medications. Physical examination reveals a pleasant,
pale adolescent male with faint systolic murmur. Laboratory
testing highly suggests a new diagnosis of acute leukemia.
The patient's parents find you outside of his examination
room and ask for results. "Doctor, is it something bad? If it is,
you can let us know but please don't tell him. He's had a hard
time adjusting after our move and any more bad news would
crush him. Can we wait a few weeks or months?"

What do you do now?

CONSENT, DISSENT, AND ASSENT IN CARE OF MINORS IN THE EMERGENCY DEPARTMENT

This case describes the presentation of a 12-year-old patient who is diagnosed with acute leukemia. Having newly moved to the area, he has no established primary care physician with whom to partner in relaying the diagnosis to the patient and family. His family asks you, in confidence, to spare their child any bad news but instead to solely relay the diagnosis to them.

Many ethical dilemmas relate to the presentation of minors to emergency care. In order to fully understand the situation outlined, it is important to address some foundational concepts in the provision of medical care to minors. In an ideal situation, minors presenting to the emergency department for care are accompanied by at least one parent or legal guardian; all parties are present and in agreement with the evaluation and treatments recommended by the physician. In the text that follows, we outline some scenarios in which less-than-ideal situations occur and the legally and ethically sound ways in which an emergency physician can move forward.

Assent by a Minor

Recently, there has been a shift by bioethicists to consider the right of the child to assent for his or her own care. This "assent" highlights the third of three interests in decision-making of medical care for minors, the other two being the physician's responsibility to treat the patient and the parents' or legal guardians' permission to treat a minor under their care. Inclusion of assent places an emphasis on the decision-making abilities and rights of the child, tailored to an appropriate developmental level. Regarding appropriate age to include children in the decision-making process, some studies show that children as young as 9 years have some ability to understand their situation and provide input on their medical care. However, it is important to note that there is not a recommended absolute cutoff. Inclusion of children in decision-making requires an assessment of emotional maturity and cognitive development by the physician. Furthermore, it is important to note that physicians generally underestimate children's capacity for and desire to participate in decision-making. Currently, there are no laws regarding the inclusion of children in their own decision-making, but rather, a set of recommendations that, when followed, are beneficial to the patient and family. Assent allows children to express their interests and more fully participate in their care; it is not a binding agreement but rather an ideal and a means that fosters openness with both their legal decision makers and the health care team. Generally, the opportunity for assent is easier to offer when the consequences of a decision are smaller or when minors are perceived to be making the right choice. Assent is also more easily accepted when in line with parental decisions or when the benefit of a treatment is less obvious. It is ethically permissible to provide care without a child's assent if limited by age or illness. A minor patient's assent, as well as the maturity level and understanding of the situation, should be documented in the process of delivering medical care.

Parental Dissent

Parents and legal guardians are generally assumed to make decisions that are in the best interests of their child. In cases where parents and legal guardians refuse recommended care for a minor, they are held to a minimum standard of avoiding harm as a result of the decision made. Refusals should first be addressed by the provider by exploring reasons for the refusal, goals of care, and negotiation to an acceptable compromise, if possible. As a last resort, governmental agencies may need to intervene despite parent preferences. Obvious cases in which parental refusal could be superseded include not only those involving child abuse or neglect, but also situations when parents are intoxicated or considered impaired in their decision-making.

Care of a Minor Without Parental Consent

Pediatric patients not infrequently present to the emergency department seeking care without the presence of a parent or legal guardian. Children are more commonly being supervised outside the traditional framework of family due to nontraditional family structures and dual or single parents working outside the home. Adolescent patients often present without parents for reasons related to trauma, substance use, exacerbation of chronic illnesses, and gynecologic concerns. Current state and federal laws as well as medical ethics guidelines support the treatment of minors with an emergency condition regardless of whether a parent or guardian is available for consent. Specifically, the Emergency Medical Treatment and Active Labor

Act (EMTALA) mandates that all patients presenting to the emergency department receive a medical screening examination; this is inclusive of minors, regardless of whether a parent or guardian is present. If an emergent time-sensitive condition is identified, the "doctrine of implied consent," or "emergency exception rule," assumes that a guardian would consent to treatment that is in the best interest of the child. Emergency stabilization, treatment, and transfer to definitive care are included in this rule. While providers should make every effort to contact a guardian and obtain consent (and these efforts be documented), this should not delay care. If an emergent condition is not identified during the initial medical screening, nonemergency care should generally be delayed until consent by a parent or guardian can be given, with some exceptions.

Emancipated minors are a group of minors who can give their own consent; each person who is labeled an emancipated minor possesses some characteristic indicative of independence. While the definition of emancipation varies from state to state, in general, those who serve in the military, are financially independent and live apart from parents, pregnant, or who are parents themselves can be considered part of this cohort. *Mature minors* are another category who can consent for their own care; they are 14 years or older (although in some states as young as 12 years) and are considered to have the capacity to understand the risks, benefits, and treatment options of their medical condition. In taking into account the consent of a mature minor, it is important for the emergency physician to consider the impact of illness acuity and severity on the minor's decision-making. Finally, although the designation of "mature minor" varies from state to state, all adolescents have authority to consent for treatment involving sexual activity, substance use, and mental health.

CASE RESOLUTION

In the case outlined, the parents express concern that their child would not emotionally be able to withstand the challenge of hearing a life-threatening diagnosis. It is important to note that they are not refusing care, but rather they are requesting that either the first steps of that care not be disclosed to their adolescent son, or that treatment be delayed until they deem him ready to receive the news of his diagnosis. Within the framework discussed, it would be beneficial for the patient to be aware of his diagnosis, and parental permission should be sought to involve the patient in his medical care, making clear that it would be beneficial to the patient and the family to be open and honest regarding his diagnosis and treatment.

KEY POINTS TO REMEMBER

- EMTALA mandates that all minors presenting to the emergency department receive a medical screening examination and, if necessary, emergency treatment even if a parent is not present to give consent.
- The designation of emancipated minor and mature minor varies from state to state; these patients are able to give their own consent. Minors seeking care related to sexual activity, substance use, and mental health may consent for their own care.
- Parental dissent should be addressed by exploring reasons for refusal and goals of care; if parents do not meet the minimum standard of avoiding harm to the minor under their care, governmental agencies may need to intervene as a last resort.
- Assent for care by minors considers the decision-making abilities and rights of the child and is beneficial to the patient.

Suggested Reading

Baren JM. Ethical dilemmas in the care of minors in the emergency department. *Emerg Med Clin N Am*. 2006;*24*(3):619-631.

Benjamin L, Ishimine P, Joseph M, et al. Evaluation and treatment of minors. *Ann Emerg Med*. 2018;*71*(2):225–232. https://doi.org/10.1016/j.annemergmed.2017.06.039

Cole CM, Kodish E. Minors' right to know and therapeutic privilege. *Virtual Mentor*. 2013;*15*(8):638–644. doi:10.1001/virtualmentor.2013.15.8.ecas1-1308

Committee on Pediatric Emergency Medicine. Consent for emergency medical services for children and adolescents. *Pediatrics*. 2003;*111*(3):703–706.

Committee on Pediatric Emergency Medicine and Committee on Bioethics. Policy statement—consent for emergency medical services for children and adolescents. *Pediatrics*. 2011;*128*:427–433.

Jackson MK, Burns KK, Richter MS. Confidentiality and treatment decisions of minor clients: a health professional's dilemma & policy makers challenge. *Springerplus*. 2014;*3*:320. doi:10.1186/2193-1801-3-320

Lang A, Paquette ET. Involving minors in medical decision making: understanding ethical issues in assent and refusal of care by minors. *Semin Neurol*. 2018;*38*(5):533–538.

Melzer-Lange M, Lye PS. Adolescent health care in a pediatric emergency department. *Ann Emerg Med*. 1996;*27*(5):633–637.

Rettig PJ. Can a minor refuse assent for emergency care? *Virtual Mentor*. 2012;*14*(10):763–766. doi:10.1001/virtualmentor.2012.14.10.ecas2-1210

23 Like, Comment, Post . . . Lawsuit?!

Jillian L. McGrath and Lydia M. Sahlani

You are the physician working in the emergency department (ED) and evaluate a patient who presents with a generalized rash. After taking the patient's history and performing a complete examination, you are still unsure about what may be causing the rash or how to manage the patient. There is no dermatologist on call for you. You post the following message in a private physician Facebook group you belong to, along with a photo of the rash on the patient's torso: "27 yo female with history of bipolar disorder, super anxious about her rash, I have no clue what to do, any derm out there who can help?" You receive varying advice and decide to discharge the patient with a topical steroid. Unfortunately, the patient returns in critical condition with signs of systemic illness and is admitted to the intensive care unit (ICU). Your hospital attorney is alerted to the case by administration and asks you about any verbal or electronic communication that you have had about the case.

What do you do now?

SOCIAL MEDIA, ELECTRONIC COMMUNICATIONS, AND RECORDING

This case highlights potential benefits and challenges of social media (SM) and electronic communication (EC) use for decision-making in clinical settings. The use of web-based applications for patient care is rapidly increasing, with little guidance on best practices to navigate this new digital medical world. While online environments allow for collaboration on complex or unique cases, SM and EC are wrought with pitfalls for clinicians. We discuss controversial issues involving professionalism, patient privacy, and legal standards for use of SM, EC, and recording in patient care.

Health care professionals must consider standards for professionalism in the use of digital content. Maintaining professionalism in the use of EC is of utmost importance in ensuring continued public trust in the medical profession and in the patient-physician relationship. The lines of professionalism have blurred as digital communications allow for collaboration via physician forums online. Such forums are often found on sites that do not have consistent oversight with regard to dissemination of protected health information (PHI), and security restrictions are variable.

This case identifies several professionalism issues. The physician should consider traditional consultation methods, whether in person or via telediagnosis, as superior to crowdsourcing the patient's diagnosis. The former options offer assurance that recommendations come from a qualified and accountable source. In this case, the physician does not disclose having obtained any consent from the patient regarding sharing an image or case presentation. Disclosing the uncertainty of the diagnosis would be prudent and obtaining consent to post in an online collaborative environment regarding the case is essential. The American College of Emergency Physicians (ACEP) policy statement on social media use states, "Verbal consent, either implicit or explicit, for such public disclosure is not adequate for a HIPAA-compliant authorization for disclosure of PHI and is not a defense or justification for such disclosures," and written consent is the standard for compliance.

Posts on a social media platform, even in collaboration with other physicians, should always be considered public and discoverable information regardless of the privacy settings employed. In this case, the physician's written word may be interpreted as biased or judgmental when disclosing history of mental illness or describing the patient as "super anxious." Further, it may portray a lack of medical competence on the physician's part ("I have no clue what to do with this patient"). Physicians and other providers should be aware that posted content may be available to the general public and may be misconstrued or misinterpreted, and the digital nature of such content allows for rapid dissemination.

Online behavior can negatively impact one's reputation among patient's colleagues and may have permanent consequences. Employing the highest standards in exchange of information on SM and EC forums is of utmost importance. Emergency medicine physicians across the educational continuum were shown to underestimate the potential for investigations resulting from SM themes of derogatory speech and alcohol use. Per the American Medical Association (AMA) code of medical ethics, when physicians see content posted by colleagues that appears unprofessional, they have a responsibility to bring that content to the attention of the individual so that he or she can remove it or take other appropriate actions. If the behavior significantly violates professional norms and the individual does not take appropriate action to resolve the situation, the physician should report the matter to appropriate authorities. In this case, the physician did post to a closed or private group but did not post anonymously or eliminate all potential patient identifiers. Unfortunately even private groups may have large memberships, and it is impossible to ensure that all of the members are vetted or control with whom they may share information from a post. Physicians and other providers should always use closed and private groups, post anonymously, and protect all patient information and identifiable features of a patient case. Despite these measures, they should always work with the assumption that all SM and EC postings are public and permanent.

Digital sharing of patient information using cellular phones or other recording devices poses significant risk to deteriorating trust in the medical profession if inappropriately utilized. When exchanging medical information with other providers online, ethical guidelines regarding confidentiality, privacy, and informed consent should be followed. Thus, identifiable patient information should be avoided in any posting online. For example, if a patient has a tattoo or jewelry included in the image posted of her torso rash, this is considered an identifiable feature, and in violation of the Health

Insurance Portability and Accountability Act of 1996 (HIPAA) standards. Other softer identifiers exist, such as patient age or comorbid conditions. Further, timing of a post or location of the online poster can be problematic, especially in high-profile cases. Obtaining formal written consent from a patient regarding photography (via cell phone or other recording device) is still standard. This information should be protected in the same manner as other items in the health care record in order to avoid HIPAA violation.

CASE RESOLUTION

Physicians and other providers must recognize that liability and regulatory concerns surround the use of EC and SM in medical contexts. This can aid in understanding and minimizing legal and professional risks. Several national guidelines and policy statements from professional societies exist to direct use of SM and EC and mitigate liability. Breaches in professionalism or privacy when using SM can, and have, resulted in significant liability leading to disciplinary action or litigation. Violations can result in penalties from employers, state medical boards, or courts of law. In this case, it is prudent for the physician to disclose all EC, including SM posts, to their legal counsel. Anything posted on SM can be considered discoverable during trial, despite privacy settings. Attorneys turn to SM use by patients, physicians, and other providers to build their respective cases. It is worth noting that there is a duty to preserve evidence that is potentially relevant to litigation proceedings. Deleting or changing EC or SM posts that may be brought to attention during litigation can violate a duty to preserve principle and trigger legal sanctions.

KEY POINTS TO REMEMBER

- Maintaining professionalism in the use of SM and EC promotes public trust in the medical profession and in the patient-physician relationship.
- Use privacy settings liberally to limit others' access.
- Identifiable patient information should be avoided in any posting online.

- Verbal consent is not adequate for a HIPAA-compliant authorization for disclosure of PHI.
- Always assume all EC and SM postings are public, permanent, and discoverable.
- Deleting or changing EC or SM posts that may be brought to attention during litigation can violate a duty to preserve principle and trigger legal sanctions.

Suggested Reading

American College of Emergency Physicians. Policy statement. Use of social media by emergency physicians. October 2018. https://www.acep.org/patient-care/policy-statements/use-of-social-media-by-emergency-physicians. Accessed April 1, 2019.

DiBianca M. Discovery and preservation of social media evidence. *Business Law Today*. September 2014. American Bar Association. https://www.americanbar.org/groups/business_law/publications/blt/2014/01/02_dibianca/. Accessed April 1, 2019.

Farnan JM, Snyder S, Worster B, et al. Online medical professionalism: patient and public relationships: Policy statement from the American College of Physicians and the Federation of State Medical Boards. *Ann Int Med*. 2013;*158*(8):620–627.

Professionalism in the use of social media. American Medical Association. 2016. https://www.ama-assn.org/delivering-care/ethics/professionalism-use-social-media. Accessed April 1, 2019.

Soares W, Shenvi C, Waller N, et al. Perceptions of unprofessional social media behavior among emergency medicine physicians. *J Grad Med Ed*. 2017;*9*(1):85–89. doi:10.4300/JGME-D-16-00203.1

24 An Industrial Accident

Chadd K. Kraus

It is Monday morning in the emergency department (ED) of
a nine-bed rural, community hospital. Emergency medical
services (EMS) reports a large industrial accident exposing
about 15 workers to an organophosphate. They will be
arriving by ambulance in 10 minutes. You are the only
emergency physician. The next nearest ED is 35 miles away,
and the nearest tertiary facility is a 45-minute helicopter
flight. There are currently four other patients in your ED,
three nurses, an inpatient pharmacist, a respiratory therapist,
a hospitalist, and an on-call surgeon. You contact hospital
authorities to activate the institution's mass casualty protocol.

On arrival of the first three patients, you recognize the
signs and symptoms of organophosphate poisoning. You
activate decontamination efforts and initiate treatment,
including intubation of two of the three patients. You
administer atropine to two and realize that with more
patients expected there are not enough respiratory supplies,
ventilators, or atropine in the hospital to care for all of them.

What do you do now?

DISASTER MANAGEMENT

Emergency physicians and EDs serve critical public health functions at all times, particularly during public health emergencies or disasters. In the case presented here, the available resources and functional capacity of the ED and hospital are overwhelmed by the needs of the disaster victims. The emergency physician appropriately activates the hospital's disaster plan, presumably including a surge capacity plan. However, even the timeliest implementation of this plan does not meet the immediate ethical quandary faced by the emergency physician. The emergency physician faces ethical dilemmas regarding how to allocate scarce resources, including medications, respiratory support equipment, and his or her own capacity to evaluate and treat multiple critically ill patients simultaneously. Public health emergencies and disasters transform standards of care into crisis standards of care.

In comparison to natural or human-initiated disasters, the role of the emergency physician in other public health emergencies is more nuanced in that with other situations, resource allocation might not be the primary concern. For example, emergency physicians might encounter sentinel cases of emerging infectious diseases or outbreaks of other infections, such as influenza, measles, or sexually transmitted infections. In these situations, emergency physicians have a role in syndromic surveillance and have an ethical responsibility, and frequently a legal obligation, to report these types of outbreaks to the appropriate authorities. In this case, the emergency physician should consider other strategies to meet the mismatch between demand and resources. For example, EMS might be diverted to other nearby EDs, particularly for those patients who are clinically stable relative to other victims of the disaster event. Other hospitals or EMS agencies could be contacted for additional atropine and other resources. Local, state, or federal stockpiles of critical medications could be mobilized. If these alternate strategies are unavailable, the emergency physician might be required to make triage decisions about allocating care and limited resources to those victims who have the greatest probability of benefitting from immediate treatment.

Finally, discussion of the unique needs of special populations such as children is beyond the scope of this chapter; however, it is important to consider the needs of these groups of patients. Liability and medicolegal concerns are to be considered but are also beyond the scope of the current discussion.

CASE RESOLUTION

In addition to traditional tenets of bioethics, the emergency physician in this case, and during other events requiring crisis standards of care, faces the dilemmas of balancing responsibilities of how to allocate scarce resources to individual patients with obligations to the community and with personal and professional autonomy. The additional ethical concepts include a duty to care, utilitarianism, equity, and a duty to steward finite resources, among others. The emergency physician has a duty to provide care to patients, but in the face of mismatched resources and needs. A utilitarian approach calls for the most good for the greatest number of patients. Crisis standards of care permit emergency physicians to allocate scarce resources to provide necessary treatments to patients most likely to benefit. The Institute of Medicine (IOM) in the report, *Crisis Standards of Care: A Systems Framework for Catastrophic Disaster Response*, recommends that "when crisis standards of care prevail . . . health care practitioners must adhere to ethical and professional norms." The seven key features of this report are (1) fairness; (2) the duty to care; (3) the duty to steward resources; (4) transparency; (5) consistency; (6) proportionality; and (7) accountability. The emergency physician in this case should focus on how to best use the available resources with the recognition that not all patients might be able to be treated.

KEY POINTS TO REMEMBER

- Public health emergencies frequently overwhelm available resources in the emergency setting.
- Crisis standards of care should adhere to professional and ethical norms.
- Some public health emergencies require ethical considerations other than resource allocation.

Suggested Reading

Barnett DJ, Taylor HA, Hodge JG, et al. Resource allocation on the frontlines of public health preparedness and response: report of a summit on legal and ethical issues. *Public Health Rep.* 2009;*124*(2):295–303.

Biddison LD, Berkowitz KA, Courtney B, et al. Ethical considerations: care of the critically ill and injured during pandemics and disasters: CHEST consensus statement. *Chest.* 2014;*146*(4, suppl):e145S–e55S.

Committee on Guidance for Establishing Crisis Standards of Care for Use in Disaster Situations; Institute of Medicine. *Crisis Standards of Care: A Systems Framework for Catastrophic Disaster Response.* Washington, DC: National Academies Press; 2012 March 21. Available from: https://www.ncbi.nlm.nih.gov/books/NBK201087/. Accessed February 2, 2020.

Courtney B, Hodge JG Jr, Task Force for Pediatric Emergency Mass Critical Care. Legal considerations during pediatric emergency mass critical care events. *Pediatr Crit Care Med.* 2011;*12*(6, suppl):S152–S156.

Domres B, Koch M, Manger A, et al. Ethics and triage. *Prehosp Disaster Med.* 2001;*16*:53–58.

Hick JL, Hanfling D, Cantrill SV. Allocating scarce resources in disasters: emergency department principles. *Ann Emerg Med.* 2012;*59*(3):177–187.

Hodge JG Jr, Hanfling D, Powell TP. Practical, ethical, and legal challenges underlying crisis standards of care. *J Law Med Ethics.* 2013;*41*(suppl 1):50–55.

Kuschner WG, Pollard JB, Ezeji-Okoye SC. Ethical triage and scarce resource allocations during public health emergencies: tenets and procedures. *Hosp Top.* 2007;*85*:16–25.

Leider JP, DeBruin D, Reynolds N, et al. Ethical guidelines for disaster response, specifically around crisis standards of care: a systematic review. *Am J Public Health.* 2017;*107*(9):e1–e9.

Lo B, Kath MH. Clinical decision making during public health emergencies: ethical considerations. *Ann Intern Med.* 2005;*143*:493–498.

McKay MP, Vaca FE, Field C, Rhodes K. Public health in the emergency department: overcoming barriers to implementation and dissemination. *Acad Emerg Med.* 2009;*16*(11):1132–1137.

Petrini C. Triage in public health emergencies: ethical issues. *Intern Emerg Med.* 2010;*5*(2):137–144.

Veatch RM. Disaster preparedness and triage: justice and the common good. *Mt Sinai J Med.* 2005;*72*(4):236–241.

25 Doctors Police Your Own Expert Witness Testimony

Robert C. Solomon

A 35-year-old man presents to the emergency department (ED) complaining of back pain, worsening for 3 days, minimally relieved with over-the-counter (OTC) analgesics. He denies injury or illness. The pain started after his weekend in the Army Reserve. He reports some difficulty urinating, first noted the morning of his ED visit.

The patient is evaluated by a nurse practitioner (NP) who documents a normal neurologic examination and muscle spasm. She prescribes rest, heat, and cyclobenzaprine. The next day, the patient returns. A second NP also documents a normal neurologic examination. She changes the muscle relaxant and adds tramadol. Four days later, after a prolonged workup in the ED, a thoracic epidural abscess is identified. Although the abscess is drained, the patient does not recover any motor function and is paraplegic and wheelchair bound.

Six months later, the patient files suit for delay in the diagnosis of spinal epidural abscess. You are approached to be an expert witness by the plaintiff's attorney.

What do you do now?

YOUR ROLE AS EXPERT WITNESS

The plaintiff's letter indicates he is seeking an expert opinion on whether the care was negligent. Knowing nothing about the case, you are naturally curious, but you are uncomfortable with the idea of testifying against a colleague. Then, you recall a cocktail-hour conversation with another physician in your specialty years ago. He had a reputation for being a "plaintiff's whore"—someone who would say anything under oath to help make a plaintiff's case. You don't want to be "that guy." But he did say one thing that stuck in your mind. Negligent care does happen, and if no doctor will testify against a colleague, patients who have been harmed and deserve to be compensated won't be.

What are the ethical principles that might guide you in this situation? The American College of Emergency Physicians has a set of guidelines on the ethical conduct of an expert witness in a medical negligence case. You find it online and peruse it.

The guidelines appeal to you: Be fair and impartial. Review all of the relevant information, excluding nothing that would influence your view of the care in either direction. Do not assume that a bad outcome must have been the result of negligent error. Carefully consider the question of whether negligent error, if present, was causative of the adverse outcome. And the cherry on top of this sundae? The expert witness must not act as an advocate for the side paying his or her fees. It is counsel's job to be the advocate.

As you read the guidelines, you are pretty sure they will give you an out. You can refer plaintiff's counsel to them and say you are bound by them. When he gets to the part about being fair and impartial, and especially not being an advocate, surely he will say, "Never mind. Thanks anyway."

The reply to your reply arrives quite promptly. To your surprise, plaintiff's counsel says you are exactly the kind of expert he is seeking. He must be convinced he has a good case—or at least he wants you to think he is convinced.

Hundreds of pages of medical record arrive electronically: ED records; documentation by nurses, NPs, physicians; laboratory reports; order sheets; reports of the interpretation of imaging studies. (You ask plaintiff's counsel for the actual images, which he subsequently sends via package delivery service on disk.) You read all of it. It fills your mind with questions: questions the documentation does not answer. There are inconsistencies. You cannot figure out what is right and wrong when the same person says two contradictory things in different parts of the chart. Some of the language seems like "boilerplate," and you wonder whether it is accurate or copied and pasted. There isn't anything that says, "Insert Dr. Smith's normal complete neurologic examination here," but neither is there anything in certain parts of the narrative that sounds like it wasn't just dictated by rote. From the records, you learn the following:

Initially, the patient is evaluated by an NP, who documents a normal neurologic examination and some spasm and tenderness of paraspinous muscles. She prescribes rest, moist heat, an OTC topical preparation such as BioFreeze, and cyclobenzaprine.

The following day, the patient returns with worsening pain. He says the topical agent helps some but lasts only an hour or so, and the cyclobenzaprine is making him feel foggy. He is once again triaged to Fast Track and is seen by a second NP, who also documents a normal neurologic examination. She changes the muscle relaxant from cyclobenzaprine to methocarbamol and adds tramadol for analgesia. No mention is made of urinary symptoms.

Four days after the initial visit, the patient returns and complains that the pain is excruciating and says he feels as though he cannot urinate. At triage, a temperature of 38.6°F is recorded. The patient is seen by the NP who had attended him at his first visit. At 8:15 pm, she orders plain radiographs of the lumbar spine after documenting a normal neurologic examination "except for some mild diffuse bilateral leg weakness that seems to be from lack of effort." She also orders a urinalysis.

At 11:00 pm, the patient is still in an examination room in Fast Track. He has received modest pain relief with ketorolac. His plain radiographs were read by the radiologist as showing "no acute osseous abnormality." The patient feels as though he has to void but cannot. The NP signs the patient out to the emergency physician working the overnight shift.

At 1:00 am, the emergency physician evaluates the patient, who rates his pain a 7, having been 10 when he arrived. The physician documents mild CVA tenderness. The nurse tells the physician that the patient could not void and had trouble walking to the bathroom. The physician determines that there is significant objective leg weakness, described as "generalized," and orders magnetic resonance imaging (MRI) of the lumbar spine. After the patient receives hydromorphone 1 mg IV, the study is then completed and read by the radiologist as negative at 2:40 am.

At 4:00 am, the physician informs the patient his MRI was normal, and the patient reports inability to feel or move his legs. The physician reexamines him and documents a "lower thoracic" sensory level and inability to perform a straight leg raise against gravity. He then orders a thoracic MRI. This is completed at 5:00 am and is interpreted as showing a spinal epidural abscess at T7–T10 with marked compression of the cord.

Neurosurgical consultation is requested. The patient is started on intravenous antibiotic therapy and taken to the operating room at 6:00. The abscess is drained. The patient subsequently does not recover any motor function in his lower extremities and is paraplegic and wheelchair bound.

You read the record over and over again. And then you ask plaintiff's counsel if there is anything else, anything at all, that he has in his possession that you should read. Has there been any discovery yet? Is there anything that counsel on either side has requested that you didn't get? He is impressed that you are being so thorough. No, that's it, except . . .

"Well, there is testimony in deposition from various people," he says. "But I want your opinion based on the medical record before I send you those transcripts." You write a preliminary opinion. You are struggling with the limitation that vexes every expert witness in a medical negligence case: you weren't there. You cannot know what the patient's actual words were. You have no way of knowing how thorough the history-taking was, whether the right questions were asked to look for worrisome symptoms. You cannot know how thorough and how skillful a neurologic examination was performed. All you have is what is on paper.

And you find yourself returning, over and over, to certain facts: the presence of fever; mention of urinary retention; something about weakness— thought at one point to represent "lack of effort," but later documented as definitely real. And you also keep returning to an omission: Nowhere in any of the ED records is there any mention of whether there was direct tenderness over the spinal column. The chart doesn't say it was present. The chart doesn't say it was absent.

All of this forces you to a discomfiting conclusion. Spinal epidural abscess should have been suspected earlier. Definitive imaging should have been performed sooner. And the patient would likely (if not certainly) have been spared permanent paraplegia. What's that phrase they use in these cases? "Within a reasonable degree of medical certainty."

And there is another crucial aspect of reviewing a case of alleged medical negligence. You are supposed to be forming and rendering an opinion on whether the care was negligent, and that means whether it failed to conform to the "standard of care." Then you find yourself suddenly brought up short: the question of whether the standard of care was met is not a question of whether a doctor managed the patient the way *you* would have. No, the standard-of-care yardstick isn't you; it's the "reasonably prudent physician in the same or similar circumstances." Now you are feeling like you have to start all over again, looking at the care that was rendered through *this* lens. It's not what the brilliant, exceptionally astute diagnostician would have done. It's not what you're pretty sure *you* would have done, looking at the case "through the retrospectoscope"—meaning you already know the diagnosis. No, you have to imagine that you are not *you*, but some hypothetical "reasonably prudent" doctor in the same specialty, making a judgment based only on what should have been known to him or her at the time.

And then you come back to fever, urinary retention, weakness. The charts from the visits have all three of these things that are considered "red flags" in patients with back pain, and yet it was not until the patient could not move his legs that the imaging study of choice was finally ordered. And this look through the reasonably prudent physician lens reinforces your conclusion: The care was negligent.

Now you must sort out when, exactly, there was enough in the record to say, "Here it is! Here is the point at which the reasonably prudent physician definitely should have ordered a thoracolumbar MRI." And, if it had been ordered at that point, the patient would have been taken to the operating room in a time frame that would have prevented the outcome of paraplegia.

You look again for symptoms, signs, dates, times—and come to the conclusion that a reasonably prudent physician should have ordered the MRI at the first visit. But then the literature says spinal epidural abscesses are not usually diagnosed at the first ED visit. You go back and reread all the entries in all the charts. You still think you would have pulled the trigger when there was mention of difficulty urinating during the first visit. But even allowing for missing that, at the very beginning of the third visit, the patient has dramatically worsening pain and a fever, and he said he could not urinate. We are now being beaten about the face and head with red flags, and yet no MRI is ordered until several hours later. The patient was unable to move his legs 8 hours after his arrival for that third visit. Two more hours later, he was in the operating room. By then, it was too late.

But how much earlier did the patient have to be diagnosed to prevent permanent paraplegia?

You feel confident that an MRI at the beginning of the third visit would have led to prompt surgical intervention. You also feel confident saying that a reasonably prudent doctor would not have taken until visit number three to make the diagnosis.

CASE RESOLUTION

You testify in deposition. Defense counsel questions you in three consecutive sessions because there was one from the insurance company representing the doctors, another representing the NPs, and a third representing the hospital.

You realize that the patient had not been seen by a doctor at all during either of the first two visits. Was this negligent in itself? Was it an error in triage? Would a more astute triage nurse have sent the patient to the part of the ED where he would have seen a doctor, who would have figured the patient must have had something bad, or he would have been sent to Fast Track? Did this "anchor" the thinking of the NPs on nonserious causes of back pain? Or, did they just miss the diagnosis because they do not have the same education and training as a physician specialist in emergency medicine?

None of the attorneys representing anyone in the case asked you those questions, but you will ponder them anyway, at great length.

Your specialty organization's guidelines have definitely accomplished one thing: they have kept you from feeling like a plaintiff's whore.

- The expert witness must be fair, impartial, and unbiased in reviewing the case and forming opinions about the care, not serving as an advocate for the side paying the fee.
- A judgment about whether the standard of care was met is based on what a reasonable and prudent physician would have done in the same or similar circumstances.
- If the standard of care was not met, that establishes medical negligence, by definition. Then, the question must be addressed of whether care that did meet the standard of care would—to a reasonable degree of medical certainty—have averted the adverse outcome (causation).
- The expert witness's opinions must be based on a thorough review of the available information about the case, including all pertinent medical records, and a review of relevant, contemporaneous medical literature.

Suggested Reading

American College of Emergency Physicians. Expert witness reaffirmation. https://www.acep.org/globalassets/uploads/uploaded-files/acep/clinical-and-practice-management/resources/medical-legal/board-approved---expert-witness-reaffirmation---6-15.pdf. Accessed September 22, 2019.

Lenzer J, Solomon RC. Hired guns: finding solutions to the expert witness quagmire. ACEP News. March 2003.

Solomon RC. Ethical issues in medical malpractice. *Emerg Med Clin North Am.* 2006;24(3):733–747.

Solomon RC. Expert witness testimony. In Marco C, Schears R (Eds.), *Ethical Dilemmas in Emergency Medicine.* New York: Cambridge University Press; 2015:217–232.

Index

Tables and figures are indicated by *t* and *f* following the page number

For the benefit of digital users, indexed terms that span two pages (e.g., 52–53) may, on occasion, appear on only one of those pages.

autonomy (*cont.*)
  and postexposure prophylaxis (PEP)
    against HIV infection, 145
  and stewardship of health care
    resources, 116–17

belligerent patients, 97–98, 101–2
  key points, 103
beneficence, 84–85
  and patient information, 7
  and postexposure prophylaxis (PEP)
    against HIV infection, 146
  and stewardship of health care
    resources, 117
best interest standard, 39
bias and belligerence, 97–98, 101–2
  key points, 103
bigotry, 97–98, 99–100, 101–2
bioethics committees, 41
Birchfield v. North Dakota, 77
Breithaupt v. Abram, 77

California, 52, 85
Cardozo, Benjamin, 18
celebrities, 98
Centers for Disease Control and Prevention
  (CDC), 138, 144–45
Centers for Medicare & Medicaid Services
  (CMS), 14
child abuse and neglect
  ethical considerations in, 69–72
  mandatory reporting of, 67–73
  sexual assault, 67–73
child sexual abuse accommodation
  syndrome (CSAAS), 71–72
children. *See* minors
Choosing Wisely campaign (ACEP),
  115, 116*t*
Code of Ethics (AMA), 70, 159
Code of Ethics for Emergency Physicians
  (ACEP), 114
Colorado, 52

"Commercial Filming of Patients in the
  Emergency Department" policy
  (ACEP), 6
communication, 47–48, 61
  Conversation Prism, 4, 5*f*
  electronic communications, 157–61
  social media, 157–61
Compassionate Care Committees, 86
compassionate dialysis, 85–86
competence, 18
confidentiality, 2–3
  filming of patients and staff, 6
  safeguards to protect, 1
"Confidentiality of Patient Information"
  policy (ACEP), 4
conflict resolution, 93–94
  cultural conflicts, 99–100, 103
  institutional conflicts, 105
  interpersonal conflicts, 105
  by negotiation or
    accommodation, 100–1
Connecticut, 85
conscientious objection, 139–40
consent
  doctrine of implied consent, 153–54
  parental, 153–54
consultants, 41
contraception, emergency, 138–39
Conversation Prism, 4, 5*f*
CSAAS (child sexual abuse accommodation
  syndrome), 71–72
cultural conflicts, 99–100, 103

DEA (Drug Enforcement
  Administration), 129
decision-making
  avoiding, resolving, and moving beyond
    impasse, 93–94
  Iserson rubric for, 12*f,* 12
  rapid, 12*f,* 12
  surrogate, 37
decision-making capacity, 18–20, 38, 99

assessment of, 17–20, 21, 99
key points, 21
deferred care, 11–13, 15
EMTALA violations, 14–15, 15t
dialysis
compassionate, 85–86
hemodialysis (HD), 85–86
disaster management, 163–65
recommendations for, 165
discrimination against physicians, 97, 101–2
key points, 103
dissemination of information. See
information sharing
dissent. See refusal of care
DNR (do not resuscitate) orders, 34–35
do not resuscitate (DNR) orders, 34–35
doctrine of implied consent, 153–54
Drug Enforcement Administration
(DEA), 129
drug-seeking behavior, 121, 122–24
key points, 124
due diligence, 61–62
due process, 77
durable power of attorney for health
care, 39–40

electronic communications, 157–60
key points, 160–61
electronic media, 4–6
emancipated minors, 154, 155
emergency contraception, 137–40
key points, 140
emergency exception rule, 153–54
emergency medical treatment
additional considerations, 92
emergency contraception, 137–40
EMTALA requirements, 13–14
ethical obligations, 92
futility care, 45–46
legal obligations, 90–91, 94
special attention, 98
special treatment, 99

Emergency Medical Treatment and Active
Labor Act (EMTALA), 11–15, 27,
84–85, 98
key points, 16, 86, 94, 95, 155
legal obligations, 90–91
requirements, 13–14, 153–54, 155
violations, 14–15, 15t, 16, 93–94, 95
"Emergency Physician Stewardship
of Finite Resources" policy
(ACEP), 115
end-stage renal disease (ESRD)
dialysis treatment strategies for
undocumented patients, 85–86
standard of care for, 85
Ethics Code Standard (APA), 70
ethics committees, 41
Ethics Consultation Service, 63
euthanasia
active, 54, 57
passive, 54, 55, 57
expert witness testimony, 167–72
guidelines for, 168, 172
key points, 173

Facebook, 157
fairness, 101–2, 117
fear and loathing, 127
Federal Patient Self-Determination
Act, 39–40
filming and recording, 6, 157–60
"Commercial Filming of Patients in
the Emergency Department" policy
(ACEP), 6
ethical considerations, 6–7
patient photographs, 1
frequent flyers and superusers, 113, 132
case presentations, 113, 131
case resolutions, 118, 132–33
key points, 118, 133–34
futile care and futility, 43–45, 49
key points, 49
legal considerations, 46